An Introduction to General Pathology

An Introduction to General Pathology

W. G. Spector

M.A., M.B., F.R.C.P., F.R.C. Path.

Professor of Pathology,
St Bartholomew's Hospital
Medical College, University of London

SECOND EDITION

CHURCHILL LIVINGSTONE
EDINBURGH LONDON AND NEW YORK 1980

CHURCHILL LIVINGSTONE
Medical Division of Longman Group Limited

Distributed in the United States of America by Churchill Livingstone Inc., 1560 Broadway, New York, N.Y. 10036, and by associated companies, branches and representatives throughout the world.

First Edition 1977
Second Edition 1980
Reprinted 1983
Reprinted 1984

ISBN 0 443 01970 3

British Library Cataloguing in Publication Data
Spector, Walter Graham
　An Introduction to general pathology. –2nd ed.
　–(Churchill Livingstone medical texts).
　1. Pathology
　I. Title
616.07　　　RB111　　　80-49956

Printed in Hong Kong by
Yu Luen Offset Printing Factory Ltd

Preface to the Second Edition

Although this 2nd edition was prepared only two years after the appearance of the original version, alterations have been extensive. Several new chapters have been added and all the existing chapters have been revised and brought up to date. A variety of errors have been corrected.

The aim of the book and its moral remain unaltered. The aim is to enable students to learn general pathology by understanding it and to do so as painlessly as possible.

The moral of the book, which is also the key to the understanding of disease, is that pathology is a by-product of evolution, a footnote to the history of natural selection.

London, 1980   W.G.S

Preface to the First Edition

This book is intended primarily for students of Medicine, Dentistry and Veterinary Science; it should also prove useful to workers in all branches of science who wish to learn about the essential disease processes.

Although relatively short, the book contains enough information to enable its readers to reach a satisfactory standard of knowledge of general pathology in all qualifying examinations of which the subject forms part. This includes the M.B. examination of English Universities or its overseas equivalents or its counterparts in dentistry and veterinary science. It also contains enough information to do so with respect to the general pathology component of specialist examinations in the various branches of pathology itself.

Although the aims and general layout of the book are conventional it contains some unusual features which need explanation. The photographs which usually accompany a text of this sort have been replaced by artwork which is intended to aid comprehension. Photographs are perhaps less useful in this respect.

Throughout the book pathology is related to broader aspects of biology, especially ecology and natural selection. This is not an attempt to be fashionable but again represents an effort to make the subject more understandable.

Finally, the chapters on psychological and social pathology were thought by me to be necessary to give the reader at least an intimation of the importance of these factors as causes of disability.

London, 1976   W.G.S.

Contents

1

Understanding pathology

Pathology is the study of disease, but what is disease? It is often defined as disability, or in terms of visible changes in bodily organs, but to do this is to avoid the issue. In the normal, non-pathological state our existence depends upon thousands of adjustments which the homeostatic mechanisms of our bodies make every second, as our outside medium oscillates between over-heated rooms and cold windy streets and as our internal milieu changes from a need to conserve water due to thirst to a need to excrete water due to swallowing several pints of beer. This continuous process of monitoring and adjustment which lasts from our first to our last hours, is the substance of the science of physiology, the study of adaptation to the body's ever changing internal and external needs.

By contrast, pathology is the study of inadequate adaptation to changes in the external and internal environment. In simple terms, pathology is the scientific study of the way things go wrong.

Failure of adaptation as seen in pathology may take one of two forms. It may be a simple inability to respond adequately, for example in the face of a truly overwhelming infection for which the body has no answer. More usually, disease is partly the result of an adaptive mechanism being turned against the host instead of working to his benefit. The importance of this second type of mechanism is best illustrated by examples. Antibodies appeared in vertebrates as an aid to the destruction of harmful parasites such as bacteria. They are, however, a significant cause of disease, because if the host's tissues become in any way altered, they may be mistaken as alien and evoke a destructive antibody response as in various allergic maladies.

The major killing disease of Western man is atheroma in which the inner part of the wall of arteries becomes infiltrated by fat from the blood. This is an inevitable consequence of the fact that this part of the arterial wall normally receives its nourishment by diffusion of nutriments from the blood. If the wall incorporated tiny blood vessels the diffusion process would be unnecessary but the artery would be too weak to withstand the force of the blood pressure.

1

As Table 1.1 shows cancer too, is a major cause of death. If the organs of the body contained no stem cells capable of mitotic division, cancer would be rare, but if there were no stem cells, cell renewal would be impossible and our life span would be enormously shortened.

Thrombosis allies itself with atheroma as a major cause of death and its essence is the formation of clumps of blood platelets. One might then ask why natural selection has not eliminated platelet clumping. The answer is that the aggregation of these little blood cells is one of the most important bodily devices for the arrest of bleeding. Any mutants not able to produce platelets or to clump them would quickly die. In this instance, as in the other examples, fatal pathology is an unfortunate but inevitable consequence of a process essential for life.

This stress on disease as the other side of the coin of survival is deliberate. The main conceptual problem which medical students encounter in pathology is in attempting to reconcile opposites, such as the dual role of antibodies in defending and attacking the body. If it is accepted in advance that this duality is the hallmark of most disease processes, the subject becomes much easier to understand. The reason for the double-edged nature of many survival mechanisms is because natural selection can act only on individuals young enough to reproduce. What happens to such individuals in later life cannot be influenced by natural selection. So the young have antibodies against bacteria while in middle age antibodies cause thyroid disease and rheumatoid arthritis. The young are saved from haemorrhage by having sticky platelets which in middle age may kill them by causing coronary thrombosis.

Table 1.1 The major causes of death in England and Wales in 1977*

Total deaths	576000
Ischaemic heart disease	155000
Cancer	125000
Cerebro-vascular disease	80000
Other heart disease	50000
Pneumonia	48000
Chronic bronchitis	22000
Accidental injury	20000
Kidney disease	8000
Neurological disease	6000
Diabetes mellitus	5000
Suicide	4000
Infectious disease (including tuberculosis)	3000

*From the Office of Population Censuses and Surveys. Mortality statistics for 1977. HMSO, London

In middle age most disease consists of the unwanted side effects of homeostatic mechanisms. What ill effects nature fails to achieve, man introduces by way of environmental hazards such as cigarettes, industrial pollutants and medicines. In the young, disease is more likely to result from a straightforward aberration of nature such as failing to provide some vital enzyme.

Pathology cannot be said to have laws, as thermodynamics has laws, but it does have recurrent themes. The first, already discussed, is that disease often originates from a perversion of a survival mechanism. The second theme is that failures of adaptation tend to be self-reinforcing and progressive. In other words, once a pathological process has started 'one damn thing leads to another'. This is best seen in long lasting illness and is often due to the inappropriate triggering of homeostatic mechanisms, e.g. unwanted retention of sodium in kidney disease. A third theme is that quick bodily responses to unfavourable environmental events are often over-done. In normal circumstances if more leucocytes are needed the bone marrow produces the appropriate amount. In pathological circumstances a great excess is released from the marrow. A fourth theme is that pathological duels, e.g. between bacteria and man, tend to be fought to a draw rather than outright victory. The reason for this paradox is that natural selection favours such a conclusion for both parasite and host.

Reflection on these themes provides the beginning of a conceptual basis for pathology but still leaves the student with a bewildering variety of diseases. It may be convenient for him to consider these as belonging to one of four broad categories. This simple classification is based primarily on the bodily defect or response rather than on the causation of disease. The classification consists of inflammation, degeneration and neoplasia, and a fourth group which cuts across the other three, namely congenital or inherited disease. These terms will be defined in their appropriate place.

2

Infection: man and his symbiotes

Everybody knows that much human disease is caused by infection with micro-organisms but the relationship between man and microbe is widely misunderstood. The relationship is not one of defender (man) and invader (microbe) but rather of symbiosis, a term meaning living together. The bodily contact between man and micro-organisms is one part of the broad interdependence between species that we call ecology, defined in 1959 by Odum as the study of the function and structure of nature. It is no longer consistent with the evidence to think of man defending himself against bacterial invasion. This error arose from scientific attitudes developed in the seventeenth century and reinforced in the eighteenth and nineteenth centuries in which man was placed at the centre of natural science while the observer stood back and recorded his relationship with his environment. We are now wary of imagining the body's reaction to microbes as a gift for the preservation of man. A look at the evidence shows us that nature is impartial and that its concern is as much for bacteria and viruses as for ourselves. Germs differ from man only in the level of organisation which they exhibit. Like man, some of their reactions are protective while others appear self destructive, depending, as we shall see, on circumstances. It follows that pejorative terms such as parasitism no longer serve a useful function, merely describing a symbiotic situation in which no advantage to the host is apparent.

It is customary to speak of *pathogenic* and *non-pathogenic* organisms, the words implying a capacity to produce disease. Although bacteria do vary in this respect, the term is meaningless in a general sense since almost any organism can produce severe disease if the conditions are right and almost any pathogen can live in peaceful symbiosis in a disease-free host. A word used sometimes synonymously with pathogenicity is *virulence* but this really means that an organism has an unusual capacity to invade and damage the tissues of its host. *Infection* itself is a word used in many different ways and this reveals confusion in our concepts of the relation between man and germs in areas normally germ-free (sterile). Sometimes it means that microbes have produced overt signs of damage. Sometimes it means the mere presence of micro-organisms whether they are normally present or not. For example, the urine is normally sterile but if bacteria are present a urinary infection is diagnosed even if evidence of damage or disease is absent. Secondly, if signs of disease are present one would speak of a bacterial infection of the skin even though it was known that this part of the skin in that individual normally harboured bacteria of the same strain. Thirdly, a surgeon would think of the normal large bowel as being infected simply because of the massive bacterial flora it invariably contains.

All infection is better thought of as a variation on the theme of symbiosis. Of these alterations the most important is a change in the population of the resident microbial flora and the second most important is a deficiency in those bodily mechanisms which normally limit the type and extent of microbial co-habitation with man.

When infection occurs in the sense of micro-organisms causing demonstrable disease it is obviously important to establish which particular organism is responsible. To do this with complete certainty Koch's postulates should in theory be fulfilled. These demand that the micro-organism be obtained from the pathological lesions it is thought to have caused, that it be isolated in pure culture uncontaminated with other forms of life which might complicate the experiment, that the pure culture be injected into animals and the predicted disease develop and that the micro-organisms be isolated again from these experimentally induced lesions and be shown to be identical with those originally isolated from the human patient. However, it is not always possible to satisfy all Koch's postulates even in infections where no doubt exists as to the causative organism.

It is now appropriate to list the micro-organisms which are symbiotes of man and which may produce disease. In ascending order of complexity and degree of organisation they are as follows:

Viruses

These are very small organisms, seen only with the electron microscope. Their size ranges from 28 nm (a nm is one millionth of a mm) to 450 nm. They are composed of a core of either RNA or DNA but never both and with a protein coat called a capsid. They are obligatory intracellular symbiotes.i.e. they can only multiply within the cells of a host. They can, however, survive outside cells in a resting form for long periods even under very unfavourable conditions. They are the cause of many diseases of man ranging from smallpox to the common cold and are now widely suspected for a role in the cause of cancer.

Rickettsiae

These are larger than viruses although a subspecies, the *coxiella*, are small enough like viruses to pass through fine filters and also like viruses are resistant to heat and disinfectants. Rickettsiae contain both RNA and DNA plus proteins, resemble viruses in being obligatory intracellular symbiotes but like bacteria, are visible under the light microscope and can reproduce by binary fission, i.e. by simply dividing into two. Rickettsiae can survive for months outside the body and cause many severe diseases, notably typhus. Like viruses, they may spread disease with the aid of insect carriers, e.g. mosquitoes. *Chlamydiae* are similar to Rickettsiae but deserve special mention because they cause the important diseases, trachoma and non-specific urethritis.

Bacteria

These are larger (0.5—8 μm) and more highly organised, containing DNA, RNA, a cell wall and a complete biosynthetic, respiratory and energy-yielding apparatus. With their complex chemical structure they have the capacity to proliferate outside cells by binary fission, that is they are not obligatory intracellular symbiotes although some species, for example *Mycobacterium tuberculosis* are facultative intracellular symbiotes, that is do better inside cells than outside. Many bacteria survive in a resting form in unfavourable environmental conditions, e.g. in dust. In pathology it is traditional to divide bacteria into two broad categories of Gram positive and Gram negative on the arbitrary basis of whether they retain a Gram stain (gentian or methyl violet) after alcohol treatment (Gram positive) or whether they lose it and take up a carbol fuchsin counterstain (Gram negative). They are also subdivided by virtue of shape, e.g. the round cocci or the elongaged bacilli and in various other ways.

Mycoplasmae

These are closely allied to bacteria but less highly organised being facultative intracellular symbiotes. They can, however, like bacteria be grown on artificial cell free culture media.

Protozoa

These are highly organised but unicellular organisms of which the amoeba is the prototype. Disease producing protozoa include plasmodia (malaria) Trichomonas, Toxoplasma, Leishmania (kala-azar) trypanosomes (sleeping sickness) and entamoeba histolytica (amoebic dysentry). Protozoa are most important as causes of tropical diseases.

Fungi

These are plants devoid of roots, stem or leaf. Unlike the algae they have no chlorophyll so they are obligatory symbiotes. They reproduce by spores which germinate and send out branching hyphae. Fungi rarely produce more than superficial disease in man unless there is a major breakdown of host mechanisms which normally stabilise this form of symbiosis.

Helminths

These are worms. They may cause disease at a variety of stages of their life cycle. Their main categories are nematodes, cestodes and trematodes. The most important diseases that they cause occur in hot non-industrialised countries, e.g. schistosomiasis caused by a trematode.

Bibliography

Cruikshank R, Duguid J P, Marmion B P, Swain R H A 1973 Medical microbiology, Vol I Microbial infections, 12th edn. Churchill Livingstone, Edinburgh

Thomas C G A 1979 Medical Microbiology. 4th edn. Ballière Tindall, London

Turk D C, Porter I A 1978 A short textbook of medical microbiology. 4th edn. Hodder and Stoughton, London

3

The stabilisation and breakdown of symbiosis between man and microbes

A more conventional title for this chapter would be resistance to infection. However, although in every day terms infection means disease caused by micro-organisms, the phrase 'resistance to infection', gives, as we shall see, a misleading picture of the relationship between man and his microbial companions.

One of the many false images surrounding infection is that of man moving permanently through a cloud of dangerous germs as if the air we breathe were an aerosol of pathogenic bacteria. In fact, the microbes are present not in the air but on the surface of floors and furniture and especially on the surface of our bodies. The primary defence against invasion of the tissues by these bacteria is our intact, cornified skin. This is easily shown by a simple experiment commonly performed by nature in which children's knees are temporarily denuded of their cornified epithelium by physical injury, i.e. a graze. Such a wound may become heavily colonised by bacteria which give rise to a local tissue reaction, including the formation of pus (p. 72). Two bacterial species, *Staphylococcus aureus* and *Streptococcus pyogenes* are especially likely to participate but neither could have invaded the tissues and damaged them had the skin surface remained intact.

Apart from the mechanical barrier afforded by a tightly interlocked and cornified, stratified epithelium, the skin has at least two other mechanisms for controlling bacterial populations. There is normally a coating of long chain unsaturated fatty acids which by virtue of their chemical composition discourage the growth of all but a few species of organisms. In particular, *Str. pyogenes* is killed by exposure to them. These substances are most important where the skin is moist and poorly keratinised and rich in sweat and sebaceous glands as in areas such as the armpits. In these parts there is normally an abundant flora of bacteria of low pathogenicity, e.g. *Staph. albus* or diphtheroids. It is very likely that here, as elsewhere, these sitting tenants, by pre-empting local supplies of nutriment, discourage colonisation by bacteria which although more dangerous to the host, are less well adapted to live in the local conditions. This inhibition of the growth of new invaders may be due to the metabolic products of the resident flora. Thus poorly pathogenic streptococci may produce hydrogen peroxide which kills diphtheria bacilli. Similary, *Lactobacillus acidophilus* in the vagina ferments glycogen and raises the local acidity to such a degree as to prevent the growth of all organisms except those specially adapted to survive in such unusual conditions. A similar mechanism operates in the bowel of the new-born infant in which the growth of potentially harmful bacteria is inhibited by acidic products of the fermentation of lactose achieved by *Lactobacillus bifidus*, the local resident.

It is apparent that one of the most powerful mechanisms for preventing invasion of tissues by disease—producing organisms is competition between the various bacterial species inhabiting the area. This interesting aspect of ecology is well illustrated by the unfortunate consequences which sometimes occur after treatment of patients with antibiotics. Thus dosage with penicillin may kill off the streptococci resident in the throat and thereby allow a massive growth of fungi to occur, the latter presumably being present formerly in very small numbers only. Conversely, the deliberate 'seeding' of babies with non-pathogenic streptococci has been used with some success to prevent subsequent colonisation of the bowel by more dangerous strains. It would seem therefore that successful symbiotes, i.e. bacteria that normally live in human tissues, do not usually produce disease (to do so would destroy the host that shelters them) and by virtue of their numbers, monopoly of territory and food supply and better adaptation to the local environment are important in preventing colonisation by other strains, some of which could be highly pathogenic. This happy situation has evolved primarily for their benefit and not for that of the host although it remains a good example of symbiosis.

The population dynamics of bacteria can be governed by quite highly developed competitive mechanisms such as the colicins formed by the bacteria *Escherichia coli*. They are unusual in that they are specified by extra-chromosomal genes and they kill susceptible *E. coli* but never the strain which produces the colicin. Colicins are bactericidal by splitting off fragments from RNA in the ribosomes. The host cell is protected because of simultaneous production of a colicin inhibitor.

It has been suggested that the continual shedding of squames by the epithelium of the skin is a defensive device for keeping down the bacterial population of the skin since resident bacteria, e.g. staphylococci are shed with the squames. It seems more in accord with the evidence, e.g. the spread of skin bacteria in operating theatres, to regard such shedding as a means of disseminating germs and allowing the organisms access to fresh pastures.

Paradoxically then, while the regulation of bacterial populations by bacteria themselves always protects the host, the characteristics of host skin epithelium may either protect the patient or help to propagate bacteria.

A role even more equivocal than that of skin is played by that of the sticky mucus secreted by the cells of pulmonary bronchi. This substance kills bacteria or inhibits their growth and also acts as a mechanical trap, a kind of fly-paper, preventing access of germs to the underlying bronchial cells. When mucus secretion ceases, due to changes in the cells which produce it, a lung infection may occur. There is no doubt, therefore, that mucus secretion is a defensive mechanism against bacteria. On the other hand, small droplets of mucus coughed up into the atmosphere are one of the most effective vehicles for the spread of micro-organisms to other individuals. In this instance the mucus provides the virus or bacteria with sufficient mass to transport them to neighbouring hosts or to horizontal surfaces where they form droplet nuclei with dust. These nuclei of dust and mucus stirred up by air currents or movement are one of the most important ways in which organisms spread from person to person.

An excess of mucus secretion may promote rather than hamper bacterial growth. This is well seen in chronic bronchitis, the 'English disease' (p. 126). Patients suffering from this condition frequently develop pulmonary infection due to a variety of bacteria and it is possible that stagnation of the excess mucus may assist in this. Abnormally sticky mucus, as in the inherited disease of mucoviscidosis, also is associated with frequent severe bacterial infection of the lung. These diseases show how survival mechanisms can be turned against the host, in the first case by cigarette smoking and air pollution and in the second instance by unfavourable genetic mutation.

Like mucus, saliva is bactericidal and part of the host's strategy for controlling bacterial flora. Like mucus too, saliva helps the spread of infection, especially respiratory viruses, by acting as a vehicle propelled by coughing, sneezing and spitting.

It is obvious (see Table 3.1), that all these mechanisms involving skin, saliva and mucus respectively, not only protect the host, but also facilitate the infection of other hosts and thereby protect the micro-organisms from possible extinction. It is only when we get to the integrity of the surface cells themselves that we can speak of a protective mechanism operating solely in favour of the host. The importance of an intact cell surface is shown by the effects of viral invasion of the respiratory tract causing destruction of the cells which

Table 3.1 The double edged nature of defence mechanisms against microbial infection

Host mechanism	Survival value for host	Survival value for micro-organism
Mucus secretion	Traps and kills some bacteria	Spreads bacteria and viruses in droplets
Saliva secretion	Kills some bacteria	Spreads bacteria and viruses in droplets
Cough and sneeze reflexes	Expel bacteria from respiratory tract	Spreads bacteria and viruses
Shedding of squamous epithelium	Discards bacteria from skin	Spreads bacteria on shed squames
Acidic secretion	Prevents growth of most bacteria	Protects normal bacterial inhabitants
Intact integument of surface cells	Prevents entry of bacteria	Portal of entry for viruses via receptor sites on cells

line the trachea and bronchi. With the removal of this lining barrier, bacteria are free to invade and multiply in the lung itself. This process of bacterial infection secondary to viral destruction of bronchial lining cells has cost the lives of countless people from pneumonia.

These defensive breaches apart, the entry of pathogenic bacteria into the tissues and their subsequent multiplication depends upon factors that are often unpredictable. Viruses are more fortunate in that cells have on their surface a variety of receptor molecules as part of the normal chemical constitution of the cell wall, some of which bind specifically to corresponding receptors on the viral surface.

In the case of bacteria, a breakdown in the self-regulating population control may be a key factor in initiating infective disease. Thus, a rapidly growing virulent strain may colonise part of the body at the expense of the existing and more indolent bacterial population. This could follow a change in local conditions favouring growth of the virulent strain or their arrival in massive numbers. Natural selection would then ensure that the virulent organisms conquered. This means that the virulent organisms may be already at the site or be transported from another site. For example the *Staphylococcus aureus* may move from the nose to a surgical wound or *Pseudomonas aeruginosa* from the gut to the urinary tract. Alternatively the germ may enter the body from the environment. The environment may be the soil, as in the case of tetanus or another human being as in gonorrhoea. Transmission by way of humans is by infected patients or by carriers and the carrier is a very important vehicle. The carrier demonstrates how dangerous organisms may live in symbiosis in a disease free host. Unfortunately the importance of the carrier state is matched by our ignorance of its mechanisms. In some symbiotic systems a plausible explanation exists. For example the larvae of nemoritis are not taken up by the phagocytes (p. 17) of the moth Ephestia and thus survive in the host. If the larvae are washed in solvents to remove their fatty coat they are phagocytosed and destroyed. Here, the carrier state is presumably due to the chemical properties of the larvae. The problem in human-bacterial relationships is why some individuals should exhibit the carrier state, i.e. harbour enough organisms to infect others without themselves suffering disease, while others do not.

The carrier state is an example of stable symbiosis, at least as far as the individual carrier is concerned. Some viruses, however, may be carried in this harmless fashion in apparently stable symbiosis and then emerge to produce disease in the individual in which they live. The classical example is the virus of herpes zoster (shingles), which lives in symbiosis for many years and may then proliferate, destroy cells and cause the unpleasant condition with which it is associated.

Bibliography

Mims C A 1977 The Pathogenesis of Infectious Disease. Academic Press, London
Read C P 1970 Parasitism and symbiology. Ronald Press Co, New York

4

Microbial factors in symbiosis and disease

Once established by whatever means, a variety of methods are available for a disease-producing bacterium to express its virulence, i.e. break down symbiosis and damage the host. For example pneumococci, which cause lobar pneumonia and other serious infections, may shed parts of their substance to mop up antibody which might otherwise destroy the whole bacillus (p. 27). Other pneumococci have slippery surfaces which prevent their uptake by host phagocytes (p. 17) a situation akin to the larva and the moth quoted earlier. Other bacteria, e.g. streptococci and staphylococci produce substances (leucocidins) which kill these phagocytes.

Leucocidins are examples of bacterial toxins and as a group, toxins play an important part in virulence. Most bacteria, it is true, must multiply in the tissues to cause damage, but others need only gain a foothold and produce toxins to cause a harmful effect. It is customary to classify them as exotoxins or endotoxins depending on whether the substance is secreted externally or remains part of the organism.

The true classical exotoxins are produced by the bacteria that cause tetanus and diphtheria. In other potentially lethal infections due, e.g. to streptococci and staphylococci, toxins play a secondary role. The virulence of diphtheria is governed largely be the degree of toxin production and this in turn depends on many subtle factors. The gravis strain is more harmful than the mitis variety and this is partly because the relatively high iron content of human tissues inhibits toxin production by mitis organisms but not by gravis bacteria. The gravis strain grows more quickly in a high iron environment and so forms a thick layer, the outermost organisms being protected from the high iron concentration of the host, the iron being removed by the inner-most layers. From the viewpoint of the diphtheria bacillus, the gravis strain is successfully adapted to survive in human hosts. Toxin production, however, is not really part of the survival mechanism, and death of the host is an accidental by-product. The diphtheria organism uses iron to make cytochrome b from porphyrin and protein that it syntheses. It is only in iron-deficient environments that this pathway

13

is diverted to toxin production. Thus too much iron prevents bacterial growth and hinders toxin production whereas an iron concentration barely sufficient to sustain growth of the gravis strain diverts the organism to toxin production. In the case of *Shigella dysenteriae* which may cause food poisoning and paralysis, an excess of iron hampers production of the nerve toxin because an amount of iron above that required for cytochrome synthesis inhibits the formation of toxin. Here we have an example of a single host factor (iron concentration) affecting a single bacterial factor by two different mechanisms.

Toxin production by diphtheria organisms is governed by another mechanism, namely bacteriophage. Bacteriophage is a virus which is a symbiote of bacteria, and what bacteria are to man bacteriophage is to bacteria. Most bacteriophage destroys bacteria (lysis) when the appropriate strains meet, but sometimes the two co-exist, this being attributed to a temperate bacteriophage and to production by the host cell of a repressor substance which prevents lysis. Bacteria may be changed by temperate phage inserting their DNA into host bacterial DNA, the phage then being known as prophage. When a non-toxin producing variety of diphtheria bacterium is infected by an appropriate temperate bacteriophage, the host organism may be changed to a toxin producing strain, the process of lysogenic conversion being attributable to a DNA transplant from the phage. If the bacterial cell suffers some form of injury the repressor substance is weakened and the phage is 'induced' and becomes lysogenic. The host cell is then destroyed and a mixture of phage and host DNA is liberated. This mixture may be incorporated into a mature phage particle which may then infect a new host bacterium. The new host then receives not only phage genes but also bacterial genes from another, and possibly somewhat different bacterium, thereby undergoing a non-sexual genetic exchange and possibly acquiring new and important characteristics, e.g. resistance to antibiotics. Lysogenic conversion to toxin production may occur also in staphylococci and streptococci. It is this kind of natural genetic engineering which has made scientists wary of inducing genetic change in bacteria in the laboratory.

That bacterial toxins damage or kill body cells and interfere with cell metabolism is obvious, but little is known of how they do so. Some toxins are enzymes which digest chemical constituents of cells, cell membranes being particularly susceptible to bacterial phospholipases. Other toxins, e.g. from clostridia, are actually converted to a harmful form from an innocuous precursor by action of a host protease, a fact hard to reconcile with a teleological view of the relationships between men and microbes. The lethal effect of diphtheria toxin appears to be related to its ability to inhibit protein synthesis in host cells. Cholera toxin induces uncontrollable diarrhoea by stimulating the enzyme adenyl cyclase in the wall of the bowel. The problem in determining how bacteria damage tissues is the separation of cause and effect. Thus exposure to a toxin may rapidly lead to a particular change, e.g. alteration of mitochondrial ultrastructure as seen with the electron microscope. The phenomenon could represent the primary action of the toxin or could itself be the result of other effects even earlier and as yet undetected. Another problem is the different results obtained in the whole animal, in isolated tissue cells and in broken-up cells. Thus antitoxin (p. 32) prevents diphtheria toxin from interfering with protein synthesis in isolated cells but has no effect when cell-free systems are used. In other words the antitoxin appears to stop the toxin from penetrating the cell. In the whole animal, however, the main action of the antitoxin appears to be to facilitate ingestion of toxin by leucocytes and therby prevent the toxin from reaching vital parts, such as the heart muscle. Undoubtedly, one of the main dangers of bacterial toxin to the host is the small amount needed to kill. Even those who survive an attack of tetanus, are not immune to a second attack because the amount needed to kill the patient is less than that needed to produce immunity (p. 27).

Because the problem is closely related to the information explosion in molecular biology, the mode of attack of viruses is better understood than that of bacteria. The specific infectivity of a particular virus for a particular cell type, which is a characteristic feature of viral infections (e.g. polio virus and nerve cells, smallpox virus and skin cells) is due to the presence on host cells of receptors which fit neatly into the protein coat of the virus. This protein coat may be an enzyme and it is a general and vital part of all biological systems that enzymes fit very tightly and specifically with their appropriate substrates by virtue of complementary steric configuration. The process whereby viruses attach themselves to susceptible cells is known as adsorption. Following adsorption, the virus penetrates the cell wall (*penetration*) the essential element being the entry into the cell of the viral DNA or RNA. Inside the cell, the protein coat capsid of the virus is removed (*stripping*), sometimes obligingly by host cell enzymes. The naked nucleic acid core, now safely within the cell, is ready to begin the rapid synthesis of more virus. The viral nucleic acid begins its takeover very quickly and within 1 to 2 hours it is being synthesised in the cell as a result of new transcription from the invading viral DNA (or RNA polymerase in the case of RNA viruses). This process too may be accelerated by host cell polymerase. The outcome of this activity is the synthesis of new RNA templates which direct the formation of new enzymes, including DNA polymerase in the case of DNA viruses. Thus viral DNA, RNA, coat proteins, enzymes or lipids are synthesised within the host cell (the stage of *synthesis*). From these components are assembled within the host cell the new virus particles (*maturation*). Because of the total disruption of its own metabolic process the cell ruptures and releases newly assembled virus (the *release* phase). In the whole of nature it would be hard to find a more economical and efficient mechanism.

Efficiency and economy in this case relate to the virus rather than its host, since the infected cell is generally destroyed during the process outlined above. In tissue culture infected cells round up and float off the surface to which they were attached. In the body, before the cells show signs of disintegration, they often exhibit inclusion bodies, i.e. areas in the cytoplasm or nucleus with abnormal staining properties. These bodies have been shown to be the site of viral synthesis in the cell. The precise way in which viral invasion kills cells varies somewhat. In general, rather more is involved than a simple takeover of cell metabolism with consequent 'running down' of the latter. Polio virus for example shuts down RNA synthesis in the cell within minutes of infection, probably by coding the production of a viral protein that inhibits the enzyme responsible for the synthesis. Polio virus also initiates the synthesis of viral capsid proteins which are lethal for the cell even before inhibition of RNA synthesis could be effective. Many other viruses, e.g. adenovirus and herpes, produce cytotoxic proteins during the early stages of viral synthesis which lead to the cessation of various vital cell activities such as the maintenance of normal membrane permeability.

A particular virus may therefore kill a particular cell by a variety of uncomfortably efficient methods. Fortunately, at least one of the proteins they induce the cell to synthesise, namely, interferon, is a potent anti-viral agent, and may play a major role in terminating viral infection. So on this occasion the duality of response so typical of pathology favours the host rather than the infecting symbiote.

Viruses have effects on cells other than simple killing. They cause them to fuse and thereby facilitate passage of virus from cell to cell. They also lead to cell transformation, an ambiguous sounding term with a specific relevance to cancer which will be dealt with in a later chapter (p. 247).

Bibliography

Cruickshank R. Duguid J P, Marmion B P, Swain RHA 1973 Medical microbiology, Vol I Microbial infections, 12th edn. Churchill Livingstone, Edinburgh

Burke DC, Russell W C (eds) 1975 Control processes in virus multiplication. Cambridge University Press, Cambridge

Weinberg E 1975 Nutritional immunity. Bioscience 25: 314

5

Phagocytosis

In Chapter 3 we discussed some of those bodily properties which without being directed against any specific microbe, helped to prevent an unfavourable trend in symbiotic relationships. These strategems are known collectively as non-specific immunity. During the process of evolution there has also developed a more refined system for achieving the same end. This system is called specific immunity. It is specific because some degree of special recognition is always involved and sometimes the immunity may not extend beyond the particular bacterium or virus which elicited it. Its existence has given rise to the massive scientific enterprise, or perhaps one should say industry, of immunology.

The study of specific immunity began with the observation that people who survived certain diseases, such as smallpox, never suffered a second attack, i.e. they were immune to that particular disease while remaining susceptible to other diseases. The observation that certain illnesses produced some kind of antidote to the malady in question long antedated the discovery of bacteria and of their association with disease.

Specific immunity involves both body cells and body fluids. The cellular element consists of lymphocytes whose role is described later (p. 37) and phagocytes. Phagocytosis is the ingestion of particulate matter, especially bacteria, into the cytoplasm of cells. As can be learned from study of the humble amoeba, phagocytosis is a fairly general property of cells. In practice only two kinds of cell in the human body are truly and avidly phagocytic. These professional phagocytes are the polymorphonuclear leucocyte and the macrophage. These cells will ingest alien particles in the total absence of any previous contact with the particles but their ability to undertake phagocytosis is greatly improved by the presence of chemical substances (antibodies) which the body has produced as a result of such contact. The augmentation of cellular uptake by antibody specific for the particular particle is the main justification for describing phagocytosis as part of specific as opposed to non-specific immunity. The

17

process whereby substances improve phagocytosis is called opsonisation. Opsonisation is vital in host defence and is the most important function of antibody. The process consists of the opsonin molecule attaching itself both to the phagocyte surface and to the bacterium, thereby acting as a kind of glue. This is important because a firm attachment of the bacterium to the cell surface must precede its ingestion; such attachment is always the initial stage of phagocytosis. The surface of professional phagocytes has two special binding sites or receptors for opsonins. One is the Fc receptor which binds the IgG and IgM antibodies (p. 27) and the other is the C3 receptor which attaches to part of the C3 component of complement (p. 28), which like IgG acts as an opsonin.

There is no known disease in which phagocytosis itself is defective. Whenever there is a defect in the host leading to failure to ingest bacteria, the fault invariably lies in the opsonisation system.

The polymorphonuclear leucocytes (granulocytes)
These cells are formed in the bone marrow and depending on the staining properties of the granules (lysosomes) in their cytoplasm are classified as neutrophil, eosinophil, or basophil. The neutrophil is the only variety of major importance as a phagocyte. It has lost the capacity for mitotic division and is the end product of a sequence of division and maturation in precursor cells, of which the earliest recognisable form is the myeloblast, itself derived from a bone marrow stem cell. The mature polymorphonuclear leucocyte (polymorph) has a characteristic multi-lobed nucleus from which its name is derived. The cell is relatively short-lived with a life span of about 9 days. It exhibits the characteristics of professional phagocytes; an adhesive cell membrane so that the cell sticks firmly to surfaces such as glass; mobility with the aid of amoeboid pseudopodia and a generous supply of lysosomes, which are cytoplasmic vesicles full of digestive enzymes.

For phagocytosis to take place the bacterium or other particle must come into contact with the leucocyte surface. The cell membrane then invaginates and two arms of cytoplasm engulf the particle so that it becomes included in the cell cytoplasm, lying in a membrane-lined vacuole (phagosome). Adjacent lysosomes then fuse with the phagosome and discharge their enzymes into it, forming a phagolysosome or secondary lysosome. This may result in death and dissolution of the bacteria or of the leucocyte itself. The process is depicted in figure 5.1.

Phagocytosis is accompanied by a burst of metabolic activity, including increased oxygen consumption, increased activity of the hexose-monophosphate shunt pathway, (an important source of cellular energy), generation of hydrogen peroxide and increased glycolysis, RNA turnover and lipid synthesis. Studies with metabolic inhibitors show that glycolysis and not oxidative respiration provides the energy for phagocytosis, an obvious advantage since leucocytes must often work in areas of low oxygen tension. Polymorphs are well supplied with glycogen as a source of glucose. Although hardy in terms of oxygen requirement, phagocytosis is readily hampered by an environment of excessive ionic strength but is dependent on certain cations, especially magnesium, as well as on a variety of factors in serum. Linking the observed events of phagocytosis with the associated biochemical changes involves some mental gymnastics. It is known that phagocytosis occurs unimpeded in the absence of oxygen. The actual uptake of particles can therefore be linked with the increased glycolysis and the increased lipid turnover in the cell membrane. The 2 – 3 fold rise in oxidative activity and the 10 – fold rise in hexose monophosphate shunt pathway activity are part of the subsequent intracellular killing and digestion of bacteria (p. 25).

The macrophage

Polymorphs are short-lived, disposable cells, and most of them die soon after phagocytosing bacteria even if the latter are killed and digested. The other major phagocyte, the macrophage, is a very different proposition with a capacity for long life and mitotic division. This cell, too, is derived from a bone marrow precursor and circulates in the blood as a monocyte. It will be discussed in a later section (p. 116). Regarding its phagocytic powers, however, there are no very striking differences from those described for the polymorphonuclear leucocyte. When the two cell populations are mixed, the polymorphs ingest most types of particle more quickly. Larger particles, such as tubercle

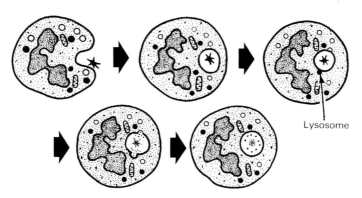

Lysosome

Fig. 5.1 Phagocytosis and digestion of a bacterium by a polymorph leucocyte.

bacilli, however, are phagocytosed by the macrophages, the poly-morphs being relatively helpless. With the partial exception of macro-phages derived from the lung, phagocytosis by macrophages is independent of oxygen but inhibited by blockage of glycolysis. The most striking difference between granulocytes and macrophages is that macrophages may survive for months or even years with phagocy-tosed material inside them, as opposed to the 'kill and be killed' technique of the polymorph. Otherwise the formation of secondary lysosomes is similar in the two cell types except that in the macrophage vesicles from the Golgi apparatus, as well as lysosomes, contribute enzymes to the phagolysosomes.

Macrophages will take up many different sorts of particle including carbon or plastic spherules. It is justifiable therefore to ask whether phagocytosis by these cells should not be considered as non-specific immunity. Two points must be made; macrophages come into contact with a wide range of tempting particles within their own host, e.g. healthy red blood corpuscles, but somehow recognise them and resist the urge to ingest them. Secondly, particles differ widely in the avidity with which they are swallowed. This is true even of the macrophages of invertebrates where antibodies, as we know them (p. 37), are not present. As an example, macrophages (haematocytes) from moth larvae were found to phagocytose sheep erythrocytes treated with a variety of chemical agents, e.g. tannic acid, whereas the same cells treated with other chemicals, e.g. sucrose, were taken up hardly at all. Sheep red cells treated with mouse antibody or aged, effete sheep red cells were ingested by mouse macrophages but not by moth macro-phages. Thus invertebrate macrophages not only exhibit specific recognition of particles, but also recognise different receptors from those recognised by mouse macrophages. In addition to this form of discrimination it is likely that fluid recognition factors, a rudimentary form of antibody (p. 37) are present in the haemolymph of insects. It is probable therefore that specific immunity in man has evolved from a more primitive form now seen in contemporary invertebrates.

The phagocytosis by macrophages of dead host cells is one of the major routes for disposal of insoluble bodily debris. In spite of its importance this latter process is not well understood, the problem being how the macrophage recognises an effete red cell from a healthy one. It is appropriate to use the red cell as an example because it is macrophages which digest dead corpuscles and make their constitu-ents available for reutilisation. Ageing may alter the surface composi-tion or diminish the net negative charge on the corpuscular surface or make the cell more rigid, all of which might lead to phagocytosis, Alternatively, the circulation may contain specific binding antibodies which attach to effete but not to healthy cells and then link the corpuscle to the macrophage for phagocytosis.

The macrophage surface has three types of receptor, Fc and C3 (p. 18) and also a 'non-specific' receptor available for objects such as denatured red cells. It can be seen, therefore, to be very fully equipped for its phagocytic role.

The mononuclear phagocyte system

If bacteria are injected into the vein of an animal they circulate briefly but then disappear from the blood. If injected subcutaneously they are removed somewhat more slowly from the affected area. If instilled into the respiratory tract, they remain for a while in the lungs and are then cleared. The same is true of the peritoneal cavity. All these statements depend of course on the bacteria not being sufficiently virulent or numerous to kill the host rapidly. The clearance of bacteria from body spaces and fluids is true also of other types of particle, colloidal carbon often being used to demonstrate the phenomenon.

This process is due to the presence in key sites of large numbers of the macrophages discussed in the preceding paragraphs. It is still customary to talk of these dispersed collections of macrophages as the reticulo-endothelial system, the name having been given for historical reasons no longer applicable. Contemporary workers in this field often prefer the term mononuclear phagocyte system, since neither reticulin (collagen fibrils found in connective tissue) or endothelium (cells lining blood vessels or lymphatics) are relevant to phagocytosis. Mononuclear phagocytes are formed in the bone marrow from a precursor cell called the promonocyte derived in turn from the haemopoetic stem cell. The promonocyte matures to a monocyte which circulates in the blood. The monocyte enters a variety of tissue compartments becoming as it does so a macrophage (Table 5.1). The transition from monocyte to macrophage is accompanied by a large increase in the phagocytic, digestive and synthetic apparatus in the cell. In particular the cytoplasm enlarges, phagosomes appear, the membrane becomes more elaborate, lysosomes become more numerous, the Golgi apparatus enlarges and rough endoplasmic reticulum develops

This process of development is due to stimulation of the monocytes and young macrophages by factors in their new environment. The cell which finally emerges is known as a stimulated macrophage. Macrophages appear as free cells in connective tissue (histiocytes), peritoneum, lung, lymph nodes, spleen and bone marrow. The Kupffer cells of the liver are macrophages. In addition, the sinusoidal lining cells of the spleen, bone marrow and lymph nodes all come within this category. Less certain members are the osteoclast of bone and the microglia of the central nervous system.

Monocytes spend about 20 to 30 hours in the blood stream. In the tissues, once transformed to macrophages, their turnover time in the normal uninjured condition is rather slow and probably they are replaced at intervals of some months. No doubt there is a good deal of variation in this respect. The mononuclear phagocyte system, as has

Table 5.1 The mononuclear phagocytic system

Bone marrow	Precursor cell ↓ Promonocyte
Blood	Monocyte
Tissues Connective tissue (histiocyte) Lymph nodes Spleen Bone marrow Liver (Küpffer cells) Peritoneum Pleura Lung ? Bone (osteoclasts) ? C.N.S. (microglia)	Macrophage

been seen, can be traced back to invertebrates. It is vital for the host because it sequesters microbes within its cells and thereby prevents them gaining access to important tissues, such as brain or heart, or achieving general release into the circulation. In addition, the cells of the system like polymorphonuclear phagocytes have developed special characteristics which enable them to kill and digest potentially harmful micro-organisms.

The killing of microbes inside phagocytes

The prevention of infectious disease due to bacteria is essentially the stabilisation of the relationship between man and micro-organisms. The most important part of the stabilisation process is undoubtedly the phagocytosis and intracellular killing of the organisms. That this statement can be made so dogmatically is due to experiments performed by nature upon man. In the disease of hypogammaglobulinaemia, antibodies (p. 27) may be almost non-existent and infections are frequent, but in the disease of agranulocytosis, where polymorphonuclear leucocytes are virtually absent but antibodies normal, infections are even more frequent, more severe and more often fatal. It seems that inside the body micro-organisms are seldom killed in any way other than by bactericidal action inside the cytoplasm of granulocytes and macrophages. In spite of this, knowledge of the bactericidal process is far from complete.

The salient facts are that micro-organisms phagocytosed by granulocytes are killed much less efficiently in the absence of oxygen or in the presence of respiratory poisons, such as cyanide; that if the post-phagocytic burst of oxygen utilisation, increased metabolic activity and hydrogen peroxide generation (p. 24) do not occur, then bacterial killing is much impaired; that if myeloperoxidase is absent, bacterial killing is seriously hindered.

Nature has once again helped to establish these facts by producing two genetically determined diseases both of which are associated with frequent bacterial infections. In the first (chronic granulomatous disease), there is a deficiency in the enzyme system (NADH oxidase is the favoured culprit) which produces the metabolic burst including the generation of hydrogen peroxide after phagocytosis; in the second, it is myeloperoxidase which is lacking. The link between metabolic activity, hydrogen peroxide and myeloperoxidase is that the H_2O_2 generated by metabolic activity oxidises an *intracellular halide*, e.g. iodide or chloride, by a reaction catalysed by *myeloperoxidase*. This oxidation releases *free iodine or hypochlorite* ions which are bactericidal.

The reaction can be written as follows;

$$AH_2 + H_2O_2 \xrightarrow{\text{myeloperoxidase}} A + 2H_2O$$

It has recently become apparent that the metabolic burst following phagocytosis has as one of its most important effects the formation of superoxide anions (O_2^-). Superoxide is an oxygen atom with an extra electron in its outer orbit. This unstable (free) radicle can either donate an electron or receive one. It is therefore highly reactive, hence its name.

Superoxide is formed from ordinary oxygen as a first step in the reduction of oxygen to water. The transformation of oxygen to superoxide depends on NADPH oxidase in the cell membrane which is activated by phagocytosis, especially when associated with opsonisation (p. 29). Superoxide is itself probably not bactericidal in real life. It does, however, readily form H_2O_2 and also causes the appearance of free halide radicles. It could also lead to the formation of bactericidal aldehydes or of free hydroxyl radicles. Its major effect on bacteria, however, is probably via H_2O_2 formation. It is eventually destroyed by the enzyme, superoxide dismutase.

The formation of superoxide and hydrogen peroxide from oxygen can be depicted as follows:

$$O:O \xrightarrow{\quad e \quad} \overset{\text{water}}{H:O:O} \qquad HO:O:H$$

$$O_2 \qquad\qquad O_2^- \qquad\qquad H_2O_2$$

oxygen   superoxide $\longrightarrow$ hydrogen peroxide

There are, other bactericidal mechanisms inside granulocytes. The *acidity* in the phagolysosomes is very high, due to accumulation of lactic acid as a result of enhanced glycolysis and this low pH (3.5—4) is lethal for some bacteria. The cells contain an enzyme, *lysozyme* capable of attacking the cell walls of living bacteria and killing them, especially if complement (p. 28) or H_2O_2 or ascorbic acid (vitamin C) are also present. The lysosomes contain *cationic proteins* such as *lactoferrin* which are lethal for some bacteria. *Hydrogen peroxide* by itself may kill bacteria with or without the help of *catalase*. Macrophages too produce superoxide anion when stimulated, although less efficiently than granulocytes. Macrophages lack myeloperoxidase but contain catalase and GSH (reduced glutathione) peroxidase, both of which could catalyse the bactericidal effects of H_2O_2 As in granulocytes, H_2O_2 and peroxidase may kill bacteria directly or by formation of free halide radicles or of aldehydes. These aldehydes would be derived from the spontaneous breakdown of unstable products of lipid peroxidation, the lipid being present in cell constituents such as membranes. These mechanisms are set out in Table 5.2.

One aspect of bacterial killing by macrophages that has been especially scrutinised is the more rapid despatch of large bacteria such as tubercle bacilli after previous contact of the host with the micro-

Table 5.2 Mechanisms of intracellular killing of micro-organisms

High acidity in phagosomes	Lactic acid accumulation due to increased glycolysis
Lysozyme	Secreted by cell
Lactoferrin	Present in lysosomes
Superoxide anion	Generated after phagocytosis
H_2O_2	Generated after phagocytosis
Catalase	Present in cell
H_2O_2 + catalase	
Aldehydes	Formed after peroxidation of cell lipids by H_2O_2
Free halide radicles	Formed from iodide or chloride in cell by H_2O_2 and myeloperoxidase or GSH peroxidase

organism in question. Thus macrophages from animals previously infected with tubercle bacilli show a greatly enhanced capacity to kill phagocytosed tubercle bacilli and are known as activated macrophages. The phenomenon is relatively non-specific in that once it has developed, the accelerated lethality extends to other comparable organisms such as Listeria monocytogenes. The basis of this augmented macrophage activity is not known for certain but it is dependent on the efforts of another cell population, the T lymphocytes (p. 38). This can be shown by transferring such lymphocytes from an animal immunised against tuberculosis to a non-immunised recipient whose macrophages thereupon kill tubercle bacilli more efficiently than they did previously.

The phagocytosis and killing of micro-organisms by macrophages in response to activation by specifically immunised T lymphocytes is one of the most important manifestations of *cell-mediated immunity*. This term means that circulating antibody plays no apparent role in the reaction concerned. By contrast, polymorphonuclear leucocytes do not participate in cell-mediated immunity but are instead aided in their phagocytic role by opsonising antibody and complement, i.e. by antibody-mediated immunity. Resistance to tuberculosis is almost entirely due to cell-mediated immunity.

In spite of being the most important defence mechanism against microbes, phagocytosis is no exception to the rule that all such mechanisms may work to the detriment of the host. Granulocytes which have phagocytosed destructive bacteria such as streptococci or staphylococci may be destroyed by them in vast numbers. Their liquified bodies accumulate at the site of bacterial invasion forming an abscess. This collection of pus involves much destruction of tissue and toxic effects on the patient and may also act as a fluid carrier spreading living bacteria to parts of the body not previously infected. An abscess is also very often painful and the patient may well feel that not only doctors, but also nature herself sometimes provides a cure that is worse than the disease.

Another consequence of phagocytosis which is harmful to the host is the secretion and liberation from the phagocyte of lysosomal enzymes. The escape of these catalysts causes cellular destruction and inflammation. The excruciating pain of gout is due to phagocytosis of urate crystals and subsequent rupture of lysosomes and discharge of their contents into the joints.

Particularly ambiguous is the relationship between macrophages and those bacteria which thrive better inside them than outside. These are called facultative intracellular organisms and include the important bacilli which cause tuberculosis, leprosy and syphilis. They are

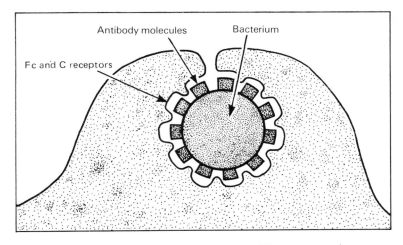

Fig. 5.2 How immunoglobulin (Fc) and complement (C) receptors on the leucocyte surface improve the efficiency of phagocytosis of bacteria which are coated by immunoglobulin and complement.

largely ignored by granulocytes and must be dealt with by macrophages. Although many are killed and digested within these cells, others survive and multiply in the cell cytoplasm and are carried by the mobile macrophage to all parts of the body, where satellite infection may be set up. In tuberculosis, this form of dissemination is a frequent cause of death if antibiotics are not available.

Bibliography

Babior B M 1978 Oxygen-dependent microbial killing by phagocytes. New England Journal of Medicine 298: 721

Van Furth R (ed) 1975 Mononuclear phagocytes in immunity, infection and pathology. Blackwell, Oxford

Zweifach BW, Grant L, McCluskey RT (eds) 1974 The inflammatory process, 2nd edn. vol 1. academic Press,

6

Immunity, antibodies and complement

The control of symbiotic relationships between mammals and micro-organisms depends largely on specific immunity which as we have seen, has cellular and fluid (humoral) components. The word 'humoral' is an historical relic and means fluid substance circulating in the blood stream. 'Humoral immunity' refers to the presence of antibodies. Antibodies are proteins produced as a result of the introduction of substances which the body recognises as foreign. Foreign substances giving rise to antibodies are known as antigens, or more recently as immunogens. The most striking thing about antigens and antibodies is their mutual specificity. The antibody which a particular antigen causes to be formed may react only with the particular chemical configuration which the antigen exhibits and with no other. If, however, other substances contain the same molecular groupings as the antigen these may react with the antibody. A bacteria is composed of many different chemical groupings so contains more than one antigen and will usually give rise to a number of antibodies of different specificity. All, however, will combine with the bacterial body so that the heterogeneity of their chemical specificity will not be obvious. Not all chemical substances are antigenic. Most antigens are proteins but even a small molecule may become antigenic if combined with a protein, the antigen then being called a haptene. In addition some carbohydrates and lipids are antigenic both in the pure state and when part of a protein molecule. It is rare for a substance of molecular weight less than 5000 daltons to be an effective antigen other than as a haptene.

The antibodies formed by antigens are plasma proteins and are known generically as immunoglobulins. There are five subgroups of immunoglobulins, IgG, IgM, IgA, IgE and IgD. The molecule consists of an Fc portion, which binds to the cell surfaces and activates complement, and the FAB portion, which contains 'light' and 'heavy' polypeptide chains and combines specifically with the antigen which elicited the immunoglobulin (Fig. 6.1). IgG is the major component in most antibody responses. IgM is of very high molecular weight

(960 000 daltons) and is often the first antibody to appear after entry of bacterial or viral antigens. It is a particularly efficient opsonin although IgG shares this property (p. 29). IgA is found mostly at the surface of mucous membranes. It has a special structure ('the secretory piece') which allows it to be secreted and is especially prominent in the gastro-intestinal tract and in salivary glands. It plays a major role in preventing infection via the intestine. It is not a good opsonin but probably works by coating bacteria and preventing their attachment to the intestinal epithelium. IgE is important in certain allergic diseases (p. 42), and plays a vital role in host defence against helminths (worms). The least understood antibody is IgD.

Complement

Complement is the historically hallowed name for a system of about 20 proteins in plasma which co-operate with ('complement') antibodies. The complement system consists of many components and is easily distinguished from antibody since unlike the latter it is quickly destroyed by moderate heating. This susceptibility to raised temperature is a characteristic of enzymes and complement is in fact a cascade of enzyme reactions culminating in the activation of an esterase which can attack and dissolve the phospholipid wall of bacteria and tissue cells.

There are three other comparable cascades important in pathology and responsible respectively for blood coagulation, kinin formation (p. 64) and fibrinolysis. When antibody combines with a bacterium or other antigen the resultant complex triggers off the cascade of reactions which constitutes activation of the complement pathway. Activated complement is also known as 'fixed' complement because all being used up, its activity in that particular sample of serum is no longer demonstrable, none being available for further antigen antibody reactions. Combination of antigen and antibody activates complement by the 'classical' pathway in which all complement components are involved. Complement can also be activated, however, by the phylogenetically older 'alternate' pathway, triggered by the presence of certain foreign particles or molecules not of an antibody nature and in which certain steps of the cascade are bypassed.

The surfaces of polymorphs and macrophages contain receptors for at least some components of complement. As a result complement is bound not only to the antibody molecule but also to the cell wall of the phagocyte and possibly also to bacteria themselves. The various components of the complement cascade have different functions. The third component (written C3) is the one involved in phagocytosis. In fact some components notably C3 and C5, split into a small portion (C3a and C5a) and a larger fragment (C3b and C5b) which have different actions. Thus C3b is the most important contribution of the complement system to opsonisation. The first and fourth components (C1 and C4) may be important in neutralising certain viruses. The final products of the cascade, C8 and 9, when activated, lyse cell or bacterial membranes.

The destructive potentiality of complement is kept in check by the elaborate nature of the cascade, by the very short life span of the individual activated components and by a system of natural inhibitors in the plasma.

Opsonisation

The most important role of the antibody/complement system is to facilitate the phagocytosis of bacteria. Patients who have all the antibodies they need but who have only a few phagocytic leucocytes quickly die of infection. The surface of undamaged bacteria often has characteristics which make phagocytosis difficult, these no doubt having evolved through natural selection. However, if IgG attaches itself to the chemical groupings of the bacterial surface by virtue of closely matching, reciprocal molecular configuration, the bacterial/antibody complex will bind easily to the leucocyte surface because of the presence on that surface of matching receptors for the free portions of the immunoglobulin molecule, the so called Fc portions seen in Figure 6.1. IgM is also an opsonin but seems more likely to adhere to the phagocyte surface by non-specific binding e.g. reduction in electrical repulsion and the formation of protein-calcium bridges. With

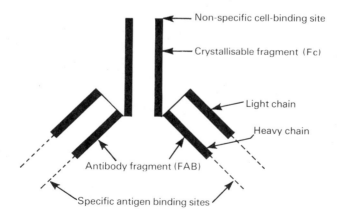

Fig. 6.1 The immunoglobulin molecule.

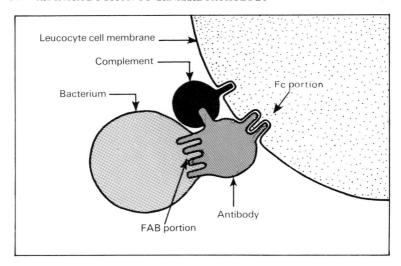

Fig. 6.2 Trapping of bacteria on leucocyte surface by antibody and complement (opsonisation).

antibody and complement bound to each other and independently to the bacterial and leucocyte surfaces, the complement system provides a 'belt and braces' mechanism for securing bacteria to the membrane of the phagocyte as shown in Figure 6.2. Opsonisation is a form of

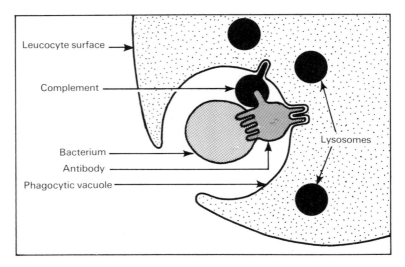

Fig. 6.3 Invagination of leucocyte cytoplasm to incorporate bacterium, antibody and complement.

specific immune adherence and it is important because once a bacteria is attached to the outer membrane of a phagocyte, it is drawn into the interior of the cell as seen in Figure 6.3 where it can be killed and digested as described in a previous chapter (p. 17). Killing and digestion depend upon the metabolic burst (p. 23) and on the discharge of the contents of lysosomes into the vacuole where the bacteria lies (p. 20) as shown in Figure 6.4. Complement plays a role here too since it will be taken in with the bacteria and may then lyse it directly or activate another enzyme; lysozyme, which has a similar effect.

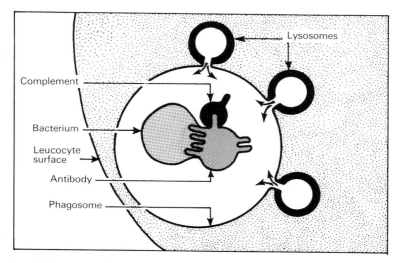

Fig. 6.4 Discharge of lysosomal contents into phagocytic vacuole.

If the host had previous contact with the type of bacteria to be phagocytosed, opsonins should be plentiful or at least rapidly provided (p. 27). However, even if there has been no such contact there are sufficient opsonins in the plasma to ensure phagocytosis. This is due to the so called natural antibody. Natural antibody may result from previous but unnoticed contact with the antigen or to chance cross-reactivity with a different antigen or may be a non-antibody substance, e.g. 'properdin' with the capacity to activate complement by the alternate pathway. When patients are found to have defective phagocytosis of bacteria it is always due to a fault in one or more of the serum factors described above rather than in the leucocytes themselves.

Other protective effects of antibodies

Antibodies may deal with bacteria by causing them to clump together (agglutinate) thereby damaging them and making them more easily phagocytosed. It is possible also that fixation of complement on the bacterial surface could lead to extracellular destruction of the micro-organisms by the activated complement esterase (C8, C9) dissolving the bacterial outer membrane.

Other antibodies combine with the soluble toxins which some bacteria produce, thus acting as antibodies to the toxin. These antibodies are known as antitoxins. Most bacterial toxins are enzymes (p. 13), and the combination of toxin and antibody leads to masking of the active sites of the enzyme and resultant inactivation. The combination may result also in an insoluble reaction product with precipitation of the antigen. A similar phenomenon can be demonstrated when antibodies are raised against enzymes which are not bacterial toxins and which are derived from plant or animal sources, e.g. uricase. The most efficient antitoxic antibodies are in the IgG group. In diseases where much of the damage to the host is caused by bacterial toxins it may be life saving to administer antitoxic antibody to the patient as part of the treatment (passive immunisation). These antibodies are produced in large quantities by administering the antigen to horses and then collecting blood from the animals. To prevent the toxin from killing the horses it is modified by chemical treatment to form a toxoid. It is now customary to give these toxoids directly to children so that they form their own antibodies, this being an example of the use of active immunisation to prevent disease, in this case diphtheria or tetanus. The protective role of the various immunoglobulins is summarised in Table 6.1.

Immunity to viral infection

The defensive response of the host to viral invasion is complex. This is not surprising because when the viruses reach harbour inside host cells it becomes impossible to attack the virus without also damaging host tissues. Fortunately viruses can sometimes be eliminated extracellularly on mucous membranes or in the blood, before major cellular colonisation has occurred. On mucous membranes, IgA, reactive to viral antigens, produced by immunisation or previous infection, will eliminate virus with the aid of activated complement. In the blood stream, IgG performs a similar function, again with the aid of complement. Viruses may also activate complement by the alternate pathway without the aid of antibody and thus precipitate their own destruction.

Once inside host cells, the virus may still be killed by IgG antibody

Table 6.1 The role of the immunoglobulin subclasses in host defence

Immunoglobulin	Modes of action	
IgA	1.	Prevents bacterial adherence to mucous membranes
	2.	Antitoxin, e.g. against cholera
	3.	Adheres to Gram negative bacilli and exposes them to action of lysozyme (with aid of complement)
	4.	Neutralises viruses on mucous membranes
IgE	1.	Attaches to and degranulates mast cells in presence of antigens, releasing factors lethal to parasites
	2.	Attaches to macrophages and binds parasites, e.g. in schistosomiasis
IgG	1.	Antitoxin
	2.	Opsonin
	3.	Neutralises viruses in blood stream
IgM	1.	Bacterial agglutination
	2.	Opsonin.

reacting to a combination of viral and host cell surface antigen. The reaction activates complement which destroys both cell and virus. Obviously, antibody-mediated immunity is most likely to be effective against viruses after a previous infection or immunisation has made specific immunoglobulin quickly available. In first infections, cell-mediated immunity is usually more important

Cell-mediated immunity
This was discussed briefly at the end of Chapter 5. By definition, it is specific immunity which does not depend upon antibody or complement but is instead due to a subtle interplay between macrophages and T lymphocytes, and largely confined to these two cell types. It is therefore easily distinguised conceptually from antibody-mediated immunity which depends upon antibody and the cells which form it (B lymphocytes and plasma cells), upon complement and on phagocytes mostly neutrophil polymorphs, but to a lesser extent macrophages. Phagocytes are involved in antibody-mediated immunity because the most important role of antibody is to facilitate phagocytosis.

As a host-defence mechanism, cell-mediated immunity is of vital importance in the killing of fungi and large bacteria such as *Mycobacterium tuberculosis*, *Listeria monocytogenes*, *Brucella abortus*, *Mycobacterium leprae* and possibly *Bordatella pertussis*. The killing of these bacteria is performed within the cytoplasm of macrophages after these large phagocytes have been non-specifically activated by specifically sensitised T cells. It is also likely that activated macrophages secrete bactericidal substances (e.g. H_2O_2 or lysozyme) into their microenvironment so that targets may be killed extracellularly. This certainly seems to be the case when T cell activated macrophages kill malignant tumour cells as described in chapter 42. The killing of fungi or yeasts such as *Candida albicans* or aspergillus is also brought about by activated macrophages intra or extracellularly.

In cell-mediated immunity to virus infection, the target is not a phagocytosed bacillus but the combination of viral and host antigens presented by the intracellular virus, especially at the cell surface. Another important difference is that in cell-mediated immunity provoked by bacteria, macrophages do the killing at the bidding of T cells. In viral infections, a special breed of 'killer' T cells themselves destroy the virus-infected cells although they may be aided by macrophages. In both cases, chemical substances (lymphokines) released by the T cells probably mediate the respective effects, i.e. there are cytotoxic lymphokines and macrophage-activating lymphokines. The most important features of antibody-mediated and cell-mediated immunity are set out in Table 6.2.

An important example of cell-mediated immunity to virus infection is provided by serum hepatitis, i.e. destruction and inflammation of the liver caused by the B hepatitis virus. This virus is by itself not destructive to the liver cells it invades and in which it proliferates; it is said therefore to be non-cytotoxic. However the cell-mediated reaction it provokes kills numerous liver cells together with their cohabiting virus. Thus the immune response not only eliminates the invader but also produces almost all the detectable manifestations of the disease, including the possibility of death from liver failure. There are many other examples of virus disease, e.g. measles or smallpox in which the unpleasant or lethal manifestations are due to the cell-mediated immune response to the viral infection. In addition the antibody-mediated viral immunity discussed above often contributes its quota of tissue damage. These are usually due to circulating complexes of viral antigen and IgG (p. 45) and the blood vessels or renal glomeruli are likely to be damaged by them. This happens in hepatitis B infections. There is however at least one antiviral defense mechanism which does not appear to be harmful to the host. This is the production by the infected cells of interferon, an antiviral host protein (Ch. 16).

Persistence of virus

There is growing evidence that a number of serious diseases hitherto of a mysterious nature, are due directly or indirectly to persistence in the body of virus which somehow eludes the immune mechanisms described above. Herpes viruses are already notorious for this propen-

Table 6.2 Effector Mechanisms of specific host immunity

Type of immunity	Target	Mechanism
Cell-mediated	Large bacteria e.g. tubercle bacillus	Intracellular killing after phagocytosis by T-cell activated macrophages
	Fungi	Extracellular killing by secretory products of T-cell activated macrophages
	Intracellular virus	Destruction by killer T cells and T-cell activated macrophages
	Helminths and Protozoa	Control of eosinophils and mast cells by sensitised T cells
Antibody-mediated	Most bacteria	Opsonisation by IgG or IgM leading to phagocytosis by polymorphs and macrophages
	Extracellular viruses	Extracellular destruction by IgM or IgG-activated complement. Destruction on mucous membranes by complement after binding by IgA
	Extracellular bacteria	Extracellular destruction by IgM or IgG-activated complement
		Destruction on mucous membranes by complement, after binding by IgA
	Helminths and Protozoa	Extracellular destruction by contents of mast cells degranulated by IgE

sity. In some cases they persist by inducing the host cell to form Fc receptors which bind and inactivate anti-herpes IgG, certainly an elegant survival mechanism for the virus if inconvenient for the patient. A slightly more elaborate device is the incorporation by the virus of the Fc and C3 immunoglobulin antigens, so that IgG is formed against these receptors, therby protecting the virus by neutralising the antibody-forming lymphocytes (B cells) on which these receptors are sited. A third mechanism is the modification by a virus of the surface antigens of helper T cells (p. 38), so that they are unable to assist in the formation of antiviral immunoglobulin by B cells. Finally, the virus may exist in cells in an 'incomplete' form, able to replicate slowly and to evade the immune response because it has evolved a form which lacks highly immunogenic antigens. Three lethal forms of brain inflammation and destruction are now thought to be due to this ingenious mechanism: subacute sclerosing panencephalitis, due to incomplete measles virus; Jakob-Creutzfeld disease, a form of pre-senile dementia and Kuru, a similar malady confined to cannibal tribes in New Guinea. As might be predicted these latter are a disappearing band.

Obviously, viral persistence can be due to a disturbance in host defence mechanism (immunodeficiency) as well as to viral ingenuity. Lack of available complement, as a result for example of genetic factors, may result in antibody merely removing viral antigen from the surface of the infected cell so that the intracellular virus becomes inviolate and therefore persists. Persistence of virus is closely linked to the development of antibodies to host tissues (auto-immunity) since the prolonged presence of viral antigen in virtual combination with host antigens leads to the formation of antibodies to the latter. This often results in auto-immune disease (p. 54). It is not always clear, as for example in type I diabetes mellitus (p. 226) whether it is the virus or the auto-antibodies which is the major cause of cellular damage. There is widespread suspicion that multiple sclerosis (p. 159) is due to the same destructive combination and much research activity is currently devoted to testing this hypothesis.

Bibliography for Chapter 6 appears on p. 57.

7

The formation of antibodies

Although it is conventional as we have seen to divide specific immunity into cellular and humoral components, antibodies which contribute the humoral element themselves owe their existence to the development of a particular cell system, the lymphoid tissue, since it is lymphocytes which manufacture the immunoglobulins. The lowest vertebrate to possess a recognisable lymphoid system is the lamprey. The complement system appeared later in evolution than the lymphoid tissue and is first recognisable in the paddle fish.

In mammals, including man, the lymphoid tissue is located in lymph nodes (also known as lymph glands) all over the body, e.g. in the neck, axilla and mesentery. Lymphoid tissue is present also in the spleen, bone marrow and intestinal wall and in small amounts in other organs, such as the lungs. The thymus gland too is part of the lymphoid system. In most instances the lymph nodes are the most important sites of antibody production. These bean-shaped organs are fed by protein-containing extravascular fluid known as lymph which arrives at the periphery of the node and is drained off at the hilum. In the substance of the lymph node the lymph filters through a network of sinusoids lined by cells of the mononuclear phagocyte system. These cells trap bacteria very efficiently and as a result lymph glands readily become inflamed during bacterial infection of the tissues draining into them. This mopping up effect, although painful, often prevents a generalised dissemination of large numbers of bacteria in the blood stream, a potentially lethal situation known as septicaemia.

It is obvious that the lymph nodes are well placed to catch antigens and therefore ideal sites for the production of antibodies. The spleen plays a similar role for antigens arriving by the blood stream as opposed to the lymph. On arrival at the node antigen is taken up by the mononuclear phagocytes and in fact most antigens need to be ingested by macrophages for antibody formation to proceed. Uptake of antigen by macrophages may indicate either conversion of antigen to a more immunogenic form or merely collection of excess antigen that might otherwise inhibit antibody formation.

The essential process in the manufacture of antibodies is the mitotic proliferation of a particular family (clone) of lymphocytes with the inherited capability to respond to a particular antigen by both proliferating and synthesising the specific antibody reacting with that antigen. These antibody-forming clones make up the B lymphocyte population of the body which resides in the lymphoid organs described above. During the process of immunoglobulin synthesis they tend to change their appearance from that of a small lymphocyte to that of a plasma cell, but the morphological transformation does not appear to be essential.

The specific proliferative response of B lymphocytes to individual antigens is known as clonal selection. The particular antigen is recognised only by those B lymphocytes capable of responding to it. Other clones ignore its presence. Recognition is achieved by the simple means of the lymphocyte having on its surface a sample of the immunoglobulin it will manufacture when the appropriate antigen arrives. Antigen and antibody sample recognise each other and this is the signal for the activated clone to proliferate and produce antibodies.

Before it can do so however it must receive another signal from another population of cells, the T lymphocytes. (see Table 7.1) These cells originate like B cells, in the bone marrow but have spent some time sequestered in the thymus gland. Having been programmed in that organ by contact with thymic epithelium they spend much of their subsequent life circulating around the body and passing through the lymphoid tissues. T lymphocytes which give the 'go-ahead' signal to B cells are known as helper cells. The nature of the signal is not yet known and it may sometimes be directed at a macrophage, which then signals the B lymphocyte, or the signal may pass directly to the B cell. The way in which T lymphocytes recognise antigens is less clear than in the case of B lymphocytes. It may be that they respond to a different part of the antigen, perhaps a less specific part, e.g. the carrier portion of the haptene (p. 27). Not all antigens require helper cells, but their existence is due presumably to evolutionary pressure to make antibody production more efficient.

There is another important sub-population of T cells known as suppressor cells. These are able to prevent B cells from multiplying and making antibody, even though the B cells have reacted with an apparently effective antibody-worthy antigen. The suppression seems to occur when the T cells recognise part of the antigen as too closely resembling a constituent of host tissue. If T suppressor cells were deficient in numbers or effectiveness it would be predicted that antibodies would arise to host tissues (auto-immunity, p. 54). This situation seems to be actual rather than hypothetical in a number of diseases. Suppressor cells also play a major role in immunological tolerance (see below).

The main conceptual difficulty with the picture of antibody production set out above is the suggestion that for every conceivable antigen which the body might encounter there is a clone of B cells, ready and waiting. There are three complementary answers to this question. The first is that a clone may have immunoglobulin on its surface which 'fits' more than one antigen. The second is that the possible chemical configurations are not in fact infinite but number a mere 10^5. The third and perhaps most convincing is that the gene in B lymphocytes which codes for the most variable portion of the immunoglobulin molecule is subject to a high rate of mutation. This means that as a clone divides, its progeny provide a much wider range of antigen recognition than that afforded by the original parent cell. This means in turn that the more antigens are responded to during the host's lifetime, the greater the potential for recognition of other antigens not yet encountered.

Table 7.1 A comparison of the main properties of T and B lymphocytes

T Cells	B Cells
Re-circulating long-lived lymphocytes	Re-circulating short-lived lymphocytes
Formed in bone marrow	Formed in bone marrow
Programmed in thymus	Not programmed in thymus
Do not form plasma cells	Form plasma cells
Do not form immunoglobulins	Form immunoglobulins
Present in paracortical areas of lymph nodes	Present in cortex and germinal centres of lymph nodes
Help or suppress immunoglobulin formation by B cells	Respond to T cell regulation
Responsible for cell-mediated immunity and hypersensitivity	Responsible for humoral (antibody) mediated-immunity and hypersensitivity
Form lymphokines	Do not form lymphokines
Do not possess Fc and C3 receptors	Possess Fc and C3 receptors

After the arrival of antigen, 10–14 days elapse before antibody is detected in the blood. This is the primary response. During the interval between introduction of antigen and appearance of antibody there is a proliferation of the appropriate clone of B cells as described above. Some of the clone proceeds to the synthesis of the appropriate antibody. Other members of the clone of B cells develop the capacity to produce the antibody but remain in latent form as memory cells. If and when the host receives a second dose of antigen, the memory cells now provide a clone of cells ready to synthesise antibody immediately. As a result a second challenge is met by a much more rapid and long-lasting antibody production (secondary response) than happens in the primary response.

The process of antibody formation in response to bacterial or viral antigen is known as active acquired immunity and may be a result of a natural infection or may be artificially induced by injecting dead organisms, as in inoculation against typhoid fever, or those modified so as to be harmless (attenuated) as in the BCG vaccine against tuberculosis, or harmless organisms of similar antigenic composition as in smallpox vaccination.

Under some circumstances entry of antigen to the lymphoid tissue leads not only to no antibody production, but to a state of unresponsiveness in which no amount of antigen succeeds in forming antibody. This state is known as tolerance, is dependent upon T lymphocytes, is easier to produce in fetal or newborn animals than in adults, is more readily demonstrated with weak than with powerful antigens and can be achieved by giving either very high or very low doses of antigen. Tolerance is a survival mechanism for mammals in the sense that the fetus develops tolerance very readily. Since almost the only antigens which reach it are derived from its own or its mothers tissues, tolerance ensures that no lymphocyte clones appear with the ability to produce antibody against the individual's own tissues. This paralysis of response against one's own chemical constituents normally lasts a lifetime. If not, auto-immune disease may develop (p. 54). Obviously, tolerance makes the fetus and newborn infant very vulnerable to infection since bacteria or viruses reaching it could be interpreted as self antigens as opposed to non-self. This situation is largely covered by the transfer of antibody from mother to fetus across the placenta or by suckling. However, if the mother is herself a carrier of a virus or bacteria, the fetus may become infected if placental infection occurs as it does with rubella virus or the treponema which causes syphilis. Alternatively, a virus may be transmitted to the fetus from the mother (vertical transmission) and lead to a carrier state in the baby or remain in its cells in latent form. Such successful transmission can be regarded as an example of a symbiote, e.g. a virus, using a host mechanism to ensure its own survival.

The mechanism of tolerance is not certain but may be due to the early formation of blocking antibody which prevents an effective response to the antigen. This antibody would be formed by tolerant B cells and would act on the surface of T cells thereby preventing them from functioning as helper cells. The most fashionable view is that the commonest cause is proliferation of a specific clone of T suppressor cells which prevents antibody formation or cell-mediated immunity.

Immunodeficiency

Nature performs experiments which although often terrible in their effects, help us to understand the mechanism and importance of phagocytosis and intracellular killing of bacteria in the control of microbiological symbiosis (p. 23). These rare diseases have their counterpart in the lymphoid system. An uncommon inherited condition called hypogammaglobulinaemia is associated with a very much diminished capacity to form immunoglobulins. As might be predicted in a primary deficiency of B cells, plasma cells and germinal centres are few and far between in the lymphoid tissue of these patients and the patients suffer from recurrent bacterial infections.

Even less common is an inherited disease in which the thymus gland and the lymphocytes dependent on it fail to develop. Affected children suffer from severe viral and fungal infections because of a lessened capacity for cellular immunity (p. 33) which is under the control of helper T cells. There is also a mixed form of inherited immunodeficiency in which there is both lack of humoral immunity, i.e. hypogammaglobulinaemia and of cellular immunity. These children show an almost complete absence of lymphoid tissue all over the body as well as a rudimentary thymus gland and die predictably at an early age after uncontrollable bacterial and viral infections. In other diseases, e.g. certain forms of cancer, both T and B lymphocyte function can be depressed as a secondary phenomenon with resultant defects in the immune response. The mechanism underlying these enfeebled reactions is unknown.

Bibliography for Chapter 7 appears on p. 57.

8

Hypersensitivity

Hypersensitivity or allergy can be defined as any immunological reaction which produces tissue damage in the reacting individual. Students often find this concept hard to understand since the word immunological implies defence of the host tissues rather than their injury. They are not helped by the term hypersensitivity which implies some kind of exaggerated response as the cause of illness or by words like allergy (other work) or anaphylaxis (reversed guarding). In fact, the immunological reactions which cause tissue damage are identical with those which destroy micro-organisms.

The conceptual difficulties provoked by this paradox disappear when it is appreciated that like other survival mechanisms, immunity can under certain circumstances work to the detriment of the host. These mechanisms evolve by natural selection and are favoured because they effectively evade a particular threat to survival. The fact that they also have disadvantages for the host will not prevent them being selected, provided that on balance they favour survival. If no immune mechanism existed, most mammals would die of bacterial or viral infections before they were old enough to reproduce themselves. Disease due to an attack by the immune mechanism on the host tissues, i.e. hypersensitivity, is far from negligible but is a small price to pay for survival of the species. The essential point to grasp is that hypersensitivity does not imply an abnormal or exaggerated immune response but merely such a response which happens to cause tissue damage in the host. All that is necessary is to accept natural selection as the imperfect force it is.

The varieties of hypersensitivity

Disease due to hypersensitivity takes a number of forms and four main types have been identified, based on the nature of the immune reaction involved. Type I accounts for asthma, hayfever, eczema and urticaria and less commonly for a generalised reaction known as anaphylaxis. Type I reactions are due to one particular immunoglobulin, IgE which has the special property of binding to cell surfaces, especially mast cells by way of its Fc portion (p. 29). Mast cells are found in large numbers in the vicinity of blood vessels. They contain lysosomal granules rich in pharmacologically active chemicals such as histamine, serotonin, slow-reacting substance and other compounds. When released, these cause contraction of smooth muscle cells, e.g. in bronchial walls and of vascular endothelial cells. As a result blood vessels become leaky, causing inflammation (p. 60) in the skin, nose or conjunctivae and the bronchi become narrowed, causing asthma. These are local effects. If the antigen is introduced into the circulation e.g. by injection of horse serum containing anti-tetanus antitoxin, there may be general circulatory collapse, pulmonary oedema (p. 176) and death. This is anaphylaxis or anaphylactic shock. Whether local or general, the effects of type I hypersensitivity are attributable to pharmacological agents released mainly from mast cells.

IgE is formed by lymphoid tissue after an initial contact with an antigen, frequently a common household contaminant like pollen, mites or animal fur, but sometimes foreign antiserum. When a second contact is made with the antigen, it combines specifically with the IgE it elicited previously, which is now coating mast cell membranes and an explosive reaction ensues in which mast cells shed their lysosomal granules and release their potent chemical agents (Fig. 8.1). In addition, the blood contains a variety of similar substances and these too give rise to manifestations of Type I hypersensitivity when they are activated by the combination of antigen and IgE on cell surfaces. The

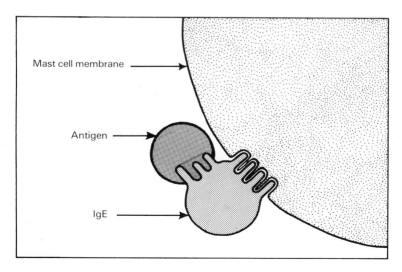

Fig. 8.1 Type I hypersensitivity.

process whereby this combination leads to such dramatic effects is not understood. Complement does not play a major role and damage to the host cell membrane is associated with entry of calcium ions. Type I hypersensitivity is characterised by a familial tendency with a variable pattern of inheritance. Those affected have high levels of circulating IgE and a stronger than average tendency to form IgE antibody in response to certain frequently encountered antigens.

The Type I immune reaction has survival value in that the contents of mast cells are lethal for various helminths which may infect the intestine. These worms cannot be dealt with by phagocytosis or complement-induced lysis so that the only immune mechanism likely to kill them is a Type I reaction leading to degranulation of mast cells. Another result of Type I reactions is the particular attraction of eosinophil granulocytes to the involved area. These may also help to kill extracellular parasites, e.g. by generating superoxide anion (p. 24). They may also inactivate mast cell products dangerous to the host.

Type I hypersensitivity depends upon antibodies elicited by antigens in the environment. In Type II (cytolytic, cytotoxic) hypersensitivity the antigens are by contrast an integral part of the surface of the host cells (Fig. 8.2). These surfaces may be rendered antigenic by ways not yet understood but in some cases at least, the appearance of antibodies is due to a drug or other chemical binding to the host tissues and thereby altering the chemical configuration the particular tissue presents to the antibody forming apparatus of the body. A chemical

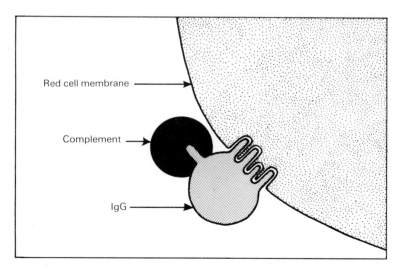

Fig. 8.2 Type II hypersensitivity.

which makes an otherwise innocuous protein antigenic, is called a haptene, and a number of useful drugs are known to have this unwelcome property. Type II reactions involve the combination of antibody with the antigen at the cell surface and usually the fixation and activation of complement (Fig. 8.3). The commonest target tissues are the red blood corpuscles and the platelets. Activation of complement leads to lysis of the membrane of these cells by complement esterase (C8, C9). When red cells are involved a haemolytic anaemia results (p. 162). One example of this is haemolytic disease of the newborn, a Type II reaction to the Rh blood group antigens on the fetal red cells. When platelets are involved as in certain drug sensitivities, bleeding or purpura result since most of the body's platelets which normally prevent spontaneous haemorrhage, may be destroyed. The antibody concerned in Type II reactions is usually IgG, but sometimes IgM.

In Type III (toxic immune complex) hypersensitivity reactions, complexes form in the circulation or on vascular basement membranes composed of antigen, immunoglobulin (IgG or IgM) and complement, the latter being bound and activated by the conglomerate molecule of antigen and antibody (Fig. 8.4). Many different antigens initiate this train of events and a variety of diseases (immune complex diseases) result from them. The classical example is known as serum sickness and follows the injection, often as a life saving measure, of serum containing antitoxin to diphtheria or tetanus. Type I reactions

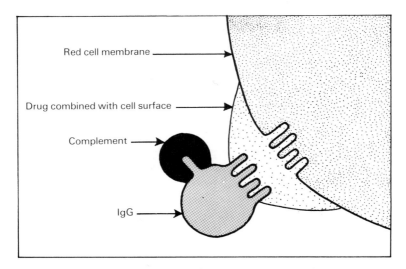

Fig. 8.3 Type II hypersensitivity in drug sensitisation.

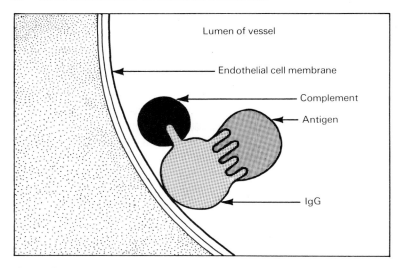

Fig. 8.4 Type III hypersensitivity.

can also follow their injection. (see above). Unfortunately, horses are used to produce these antitoxin antibodies since no human source exists. As a result their administration means giving the patient a large antigenic dose of horse immunoglobulins to which the patient forms his own antibodies. If the horse globulins are not eliminated quickly enough, they will combine in the circulation with the antibody (IgG or IgM) which the patient has formed in response to their presence.

Some of the complexes of horse protein and antibody will be removed and neutralised by phagocytosis. In other cases, however, the complexes will remain in circulation and be filtered from the blood and lodge in vulnerable parts of the circulation. The glomeruli of the kidney are a favourite site for their deposition as are the membranes of the joints. Many other antigens will induce the formation of these complexes including bacteria, notably the steptococcus, the malaria parasite, viruses, the patient's own nucleoproteins and drugs either alone or as haptenes linked to plasma protein.

The formation of soluble antigen/antibody complexes and their arrest within the walls of small blood vessels is an important mechanism in the causation of disease and seems to occur rather readily. There is a growing suspicion that many unpleasant manifestations of illness are due to the presence of these complexes, for example some of the skin eruptions, heart damage and even brain damage of severe virus infections may result not only from penetration by the virus of the cells concerned but also from formation of circulating complexes of virus and antibody. Type III hypersensitivity is the major cause of glomeru-lonephritis and the underlying mechanism of a number of less common diseases, such as systemic lupus erythematosus (SLE), in which almost any system of the body can be affected.

All the pathological effects attributable to Type III hypersensitivity are due to the same simple event. The circulating antigen/antibody complex is arrested temporarily at some point on the surface of the endothelial cells lining the small blood vessels. It breaches the endothelial barrier but is held up in the basement membrane which separates these cells from the surrounding tissues (Fig. 8.5). The complex now activates the complement which it carried into the vessel wall or which it fixed after its arrival. Enzymes are activated in the complement system which attack the basement membrane and excite an inflammatory reaction which causes further damage (p. 60). Moreover, because of disruption in the normal smooth vessel lining, platelet thrombi are deposited which lead to additional destruction (p. 140). For these reasons, immune complex deposition often causes progressive and irreversible pathology.

A very wide range of exogenous and endogenous antigens seem to be capable of causing immune complex disease. Since many of these antigens are ubiquitous it is impossible to escape the awkward question of why only a small number of unfortunates succumb in this way. It has to be presumed that most people form complexes, e.g. with invading streptococcal antigens, but then succeed in eliminating them

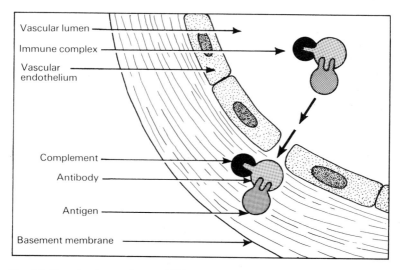

Fig. 8.5 Vascular damage in type III hypersensitivity.

without suffering diseases such as immune complex glomerulonephritis.

The answer to the question is not yet clear, but evidence is accumulating that complement plays a key role in the elimination of immune complexes as well as in producing their inflammatory consequences. Some patients with nephritis due to immune complexes have a circulating abnormal IgG (nephritic factor) which causes immune complex nephritis in animals. This abnormal IgG seems to be produced in certain genetically pre-disposed individuals in response to particular antigenic stimulation, e.g. by streptococci. It activates complement by the alternate pathway and so causes a shortage of intact complement. In this situation there is enough complement to cause tissue damage when immune complexes form and activate complement by the classical pathway. The deficiency is, however, sufficiently serious to interfere with phagocytosis of immune complexes or to prevent their extracellular solubilisation. As a result, when these complexes form they lodge wherever they can, particularly in the glomerulus of the kidney. The sequence of events outlined above can also probably arise from persistent viral infection which also tends to cause complement activation by the alternate pathway. These interactions are summarised in Figure 8.6.

In the three types of hypersensitivity just described, tissue damage begins between 15 minutes and 8 hours after antigen and antibody meet. They are therefore sometimes lumped together as immediate hypersensitivity. In Type IV hypersensitivity, a reaction is not evident

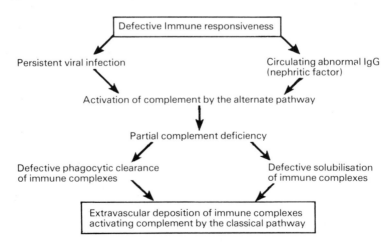

Fig. 8.6 The way in which complement deficiency, due to a faulty immune response, could lead to complement-dependent immunological tissue damage.

until 24–48 hours after a sensitised host is challenged with antigen. For this reason the Type IV reaction is known also as delayed hypersensitivity.

Types I, II and III differ from Type IV hypersensitivity in another fundamental way, in that whereas the first three types are due to the presence of circulating antibody, Type IV reactions demand the presence of sensitised lymphocytes themselves. For this reason Type IV hypersensitivity is known also as specific cell-mediated immunity (or allergy)—not to be confused with the more general term 'cellular immunity' which is used most often in relation to intracellular killing of bacteria by macrophages. The importance of lymphocytes as opposed to antibody is best illustrated by transfer experiments. Immediate hypersensitivity, i.e. Types I, II and III, can be transferred passively by injecting immunoglobulin from a sensitised animal into a normal animal, but this does not work with Type IV hypersensitivity which can only be transferred passively by injections of lymphocytes from a sensitised animal.

Type IV reactions are of great importance in pathology. This type of hypersensitivity develops readily in response to microbiological antigens, notably tubercle bacilli. As a result delayed hypersensitivity plays a significant part in the tissue destruction seen in tuberculosis. Other bacteria to which delayed hypersensitivity develops include the streptococci, the typhoid bacillus and the organism which causes brucellosis. A variety of viruses induce Type IV reactions, including those which cause measles and mumps. Many fungi also provoke Type IV hypersensitivity in man, as do insect bites, including those from the mosquito, in this case the antigen being in the insect's saliva. Drugs and chemicals may cause Type IV hypersensitivity in the skin (contact hypersensitivity). In this instance the chemical acts as a haptene (p. 27) by combining with skin protein to produce an antigen. The result is a skin rash which may be severe enough to be disastrous to the patient.

The mechanism by which Type IV reactions cause tissue destruction is not completely understood. The basis is a reaction between the antigen and circulating T cell lymphocytes, (p. 38), which have been previously sensitised to the antigen in question (Fig. 8.7). As a result of this reaction, substances called lymphokines are released from the lymphocyte. The main action of these chemicals is to attract macrophages to the site of the antigen/lymphocyte reaction and to immobilise and damage them. Lysosomal enzymes released from the injured macrophages cause tissue destruction, inflammation and further entry of macrophages (p. 116). In this way, a small number of sensitised T cells can initiate a reaction involving a much greater number of non-sensitised cells and considerable damage to tissues. A common example of such a response is the tuberculin or Mantoux reaction. A small amount of protein antigen from dead tubercle bacilli is injected into the skin. If the patient has had previous contact with the bacillus a red swelling will appear in 24—48 hours and then slowly subside. Examination of the area under a microscope shows it to be made up of macrophages and lymphocytes, some of the latter cells being demonstrably sensitised to tuberculin. Although a measure of Type IV hypersensitivity, the Mantoux test is widely used to determine immunity or susceptibility to tuberculosis, since immunity and hypersensitivity go hand in hand. If children have a negative Mantoux reaction, i.e. have no evidence of having been sensitised by previous contact with tubercle bacilli, it is usual to immunise them with BCG, a harmless strain of tubercle bacilli. There are at least two other cytotoxic mechanisms which may operate in cell mediated hypersensitivity. One is the killer T cell in which the lymphocyte itself destroys cells by release of cytotoxic lymphokines. The other, less certain, is the K cell which may be a non-T cell lymphocyte or a young macrophage and may depend on interaction with antibody to exert its lethal effect.

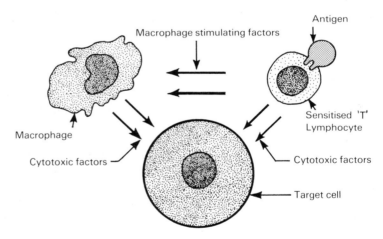

Fig. 8.7 Type IV hypersensitivity.

It would be surprising if so powerful a response as specific cell mediated immunity could have developed without having survival value for the host. In fact, the capacity of sensitised T lymphocytes after contact with antigen to arm macrophages is the basis of specific immunity to a wide variety of very dangerous micro-organisms notably those causing tuberculosis, leprosy and brucellosis. Only phagocytosis by macrophages can destroy these bacteria and it is their stimulation by specifically sensitised lymphocytes which gives them the extra power they need to do so.

A fifth type of hypersensitivity which overlaps with Type IV is granulomatous hypersensitivity. In its commonest form it is simply the contribution made by the Type IV reaction to the accumulation of macrophages and their derivatives which occurs in infectious granulomas such as tuberculosis, tuberculoid leprosy and schistosomiasis. It should be explained that a granuloma is a local accumulation of macrophages and cells derived from them and is the most important form of chronic inflammation (p. 116). In the infective granulomas listed above, delayed hypersensitivity contributes substantially to the infiltration and immobilisation of the participating macrophages and hence to the size and severity of the lesions.

The other type of granulomatous hypersensitivity is idiosyncratic in that unlike the variety just described only a proportion of individuals exposed to the antigen develop it. It is seen classically after exposure to certain rare metals, such as zirconium. It can be elicited by extremely small amounts of antigen and results in a granuloma which is slow to subside, unlike the tuberculin reaction which resolves in a week or two. This form of hypersensitivity may become increasingly important as uses are found for these rare metals in industry and in the home.

One other type of hypersensitivity deserves mention because of its importance in auto-immune disease (Ch. 9). In this variant, IgG or IgM antibodies are formed to some of the body's own secretions, e.g. intrinsic factor, combine with them and neutralise their biological activity, thereby causing diseases such as pernicious anaemia (p. 159).

The rejection of organ and tissue transplants
Skin may be grafted from one part of an individual's body to another part and thrive in its new location. This operation is performed routinely in cases of burns. However skin from one individual grafted to a different individual (an allograft or homograft) will die and be rejected within a week or so. The same is true of grafts of kidneys and other organs. Similarly, it is not normally possible to graft tissue from one species to another. This failure is due to the recipient's body recognising the grafted tissue as foreign and attacking it as it will attack invading bacteria. Indeed, a second transplant is rejected even faster than the first just as a secondary immune response to bacterial antigens is faster than the primary response.

It is now well known that the elimination of foreign tissue transplants, soon after the graft is performed, is largely due to specific cell-mediated immunity akin to Type IV hypersensitivity. T lymphocytes, in the course of their endless wanderings, circulate through the part bearing the graft, recognise its alien chemical nature and return to the lymph nodes where the sensitised cells proliferate (Fig. 8.8). These sensitised cells, now numerous, return to the graft site, react once again with the antigenic foreign transplant and release lymphokines which attract, immobilise and damage even larger numbers of macrophages thereby causing the graft to be rejected (Fig. 8.9). The role of T lymphocytes is highlighted by the inability of animals to reject allografts if their thymus gland is removed immediately after birth.

Although cell-mediated immunity is of major importance, the rejection of kidney grafts in the late stage after the reaction has been delayed by immunosuppresive therapy is due to the formation of circulating antibodies to the foreign renal antigens. This is mainly a Type II hypersensitivity reaction in which complexes of IgG or IgM and complement form on the walls of the kidney vessels and in the glomeruli. A repetitive cycle of vascular damage, platelet aggregation and more vascular destruction occurs and results in rejection of the kidney. It is possible that some of this antibody is formed within the graft bed by host lymphocytes.

The unique quality of the antigens of each individual which makes graft rejection inevitable is conferred by a set of so-called histocompatability antigens present on the surface of body cells and most easily detected on leucocytes. They are known as the HLA system or less

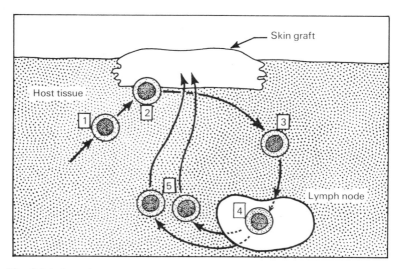

Fig. 8.8 1. Lymphocytes arrive at graft site; 2. Lymphocytes become sensitised to graft; 3. Sensitised lymphocytes return to lymph node; 4. Sensitised lymphocytes proliferate in lymph node; 5. Sensitised lymphocytes return to graft site in large numbers.

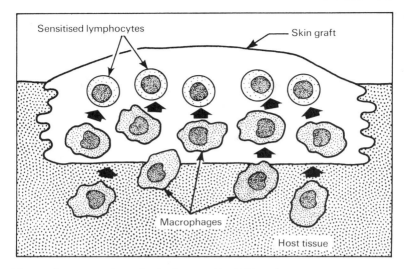

Fig. 8.9 Later events in graft rejection; sensitised T lymphocytes attract macrophages which together with cytotoxic T cells destroy the graft.

commonly as the major histocompatibility complex (MHC). Because of the growing importance of the HLA system it has been given a short section to itself (Ch. 34).

Bibliography for Chapter 8 appears on p. 57.

9

Auto-immune disease

It is plain that the capacity of vertebrates to mount an immune reaction against foreign antigens may be as harmful to the host as to any bacteria or other would-be symbiote. Nevertheless, it was part of the initial dogma of immunology that an animal could not form antibodies against its own tissues. On the other hand it was evident that were this to happen a potent disease mechanism would exist.

A glance at the previous chapter on hypersensitivity will show that in fact several examples of antibody reactions to host tissues are quoted. In Type III reactions, i.e. circulating immune complex disease, there is the disease called systemic lupus erythematosus (SLE) with host nucleoprotein as antigen. In Type II reactions against antigen that is an integral part of an intact tissue or cell there is the important example of autoallergic haemolytic anaemia. In this disease the patient's red corpuscles become coated with antibody, either IgM or IgG. This makes them more susceptible to destruction in the spleen and liver and with the participation of complement, subjects them to lysis. This shortens their survival from a normal half-life of three weeks to a span of a few days. Some cases of glomerulonephritis are probably due to fixation of antibody to antigens in glomerular basement membrane. In rheumatic fever a similar attachment of antibody to antigens in cardiac muscle and valves and pericardium may occur, causing damage to the heart. In rheumatoid arthritis, antibody might attach itself to antigens in the synovial membrane of joints and in ulcerative colitis to antigens in colonic mucous membrane. In pernicious anaemia antibodies circulate in the patient's blood which bind to and presumably damage the parietal cells of the gastric mucosa. An even higher proportion of patients with pernicious anaemia have immunoglobulins directed specifically against intrinsic factor, the protein secreted by parietal cells which is directly responsible for the absorption of red cell maturation factors. This is an example of neutralisation hypersensitivity. In Addisons's disease anti-adrenal antibodies circulate so that a similar process occurs in the adrenal gland causing deficiency of adrenal hormones. One of the best documented auto-immune diseases is Hashimoto's thyroiditis in which there is a progressive destruction of the thyroid gland associated with the presence of antibody to thyroid cells and to thyroglobulin, the hormone secreted by these cells. Other diseases of the thyroid gland are also associated with the circulating anti-thyroid immunoglobulins. It is possible that in some auto-immune disease, cell-mediated (Type IV) hypersensitivity plays a part, perhaps by facilitating antibody binding. Certainly, experimental counterparts of some of these diseases, e.g. thyroiditis, exhibit many of the features of Type IV reactions. In the human, however, they are all characterised by the existence of antibody which can be demonstrated in the serum or bound within the target organ. Blockage of pharmacological receptors on cell membranes by auto-antibody is another important pathogenic mechanism. This probably occurs in myasthenia gravis in which muscular contraction fails, leading to paralysis. The antibodies are directed against the acetylcholine receptors in striated muscle. The thymus plays an undoubted but mysterious role in this disease. It is possible that the gland produces a substance which renders the acetylcholine receptors auto-antigenic. Anti-receptor antibodies may also account for auto-immune thyrotoxicosis (over activity of the thyroid gland). In this instance the antibodies may be directed against receptors on the thyroid that would normally receive hormonal instructions from the pituitary. As a result, the thyroid escapes from pituitary control, negative feedback is prevented and the gland chemically overreacts. In some diseases the target specificity of the auto-antibody bears no obvious relationship to the disease with which it is associated. Thus in the disease of chronic hepatitis, antibodies are found directed against smooth muscle, and in another liver disease, biliary cirrhosis, against mitochondria from any organ. Little is known for certain about the pathogenesis of any of these diseases. In Type IV reactions damage could be caused by lymphocytes by the means discussed earlier. In Type II reactions the binding of antibody to gastric, thyroid or adrenal cells could prevent their normal function and lead to structural damage. Alternatively, immunoglobulin could bind to the soluble products of these cells, e.g. intrinsic factor, thyroglobulin or corticosteroids and inactivate them just as antitoxins inactivate soluble bacterial enzymes. In addition the complement cascade could be activated by the binding of antibody to tissue antigen and cause cellular mischief.

The major question is of course why the cells in these organs should for no apparent reason become antigenic to the immune apparatus of the individual in which they are sited. The answer is unknown but several suggestions are current.

T cells (p. 39) acquire the ability to recognise self antigens (p. 38) in the thymus in early life. T cells capable of recognising only self antigens probably become suppressor T cells (p. 38) and prevent B cells from forming antibodies to host tissues. These T cells and the B cells with which they interact are said to be 'tolerant' to self antigens. This population of tolerant, self-recognising, suppressor T cells is probably the main defence against auto-immunity. In other words tolerance to self antigens is an active process dependent upon proliferation of a self-recognising T cell population and suppression of potential auto-antibody forming B cells by these suppressor T cells.

Recognition of foreign or non-self antigens is not merely detecting the absence of self or the presence of something totally alien. It seems more likely that T cells only initiate an immune response when they detect that a combination of self and non-self antigens is being presented to them. Thus lymphocytes will attack virus infected cells from the same donor but will ignore similarly damaged cells from another species. It may be that some of the delay present in the immune responses in living animals is due to the time required for the alien antigens to form some kind of linkage with host tissue. On the probably valid assumption that there is a permanent population of B cells able to form antibody to self antigens, these observations make it obvious that auto-immunity can develop for one of two reasons. Either there is a general deficiency of suppressor T cells or a foreign antigen combines with self antigen in such a way as to induce T cells to allow the formation of antibodies to self alone. The drug 'Sedormid' causes the production of antibody to platelets binding it, but only as long as the drug is present. This is Type II (cytotoxic) hypersensitivity (p. 44) and is not true auto-immunity. By contrast the drug α methyldopa causes the formation of antibodies against the antigens of red cells themselves; this is auto-immunity provoked by an external chemical.

There is growing evidence that a deficient suppressor T cell population is a feature of many auto-immune diseases. It has been found in strains of mice subject to auto-immune disease and demonstrated by indirect means in at least one such disease of man, systemic lupus erthymatosus (SLE). Auto-immune haemolytic anaemia occurs in known thymus deficient states. With advancing age, suppressor T cell activity diminishes and auto-immunity becomes more common. In mice this process can be arrested by thymic transplants.

Finally, it is clear that persistent viral infection may be associated with auto-immunity. At least three auto-immune diseases of animals can be induced by inoculation of certain viruses. It is interesting, but not of course conclusive that C-type particles characteristic of these viruses have been found in patients with SLE. Viruses form intimate molecular relationships with tissue cells and it is easy to see that such a combination would be recognised as foreign plus self antigen and evoke a fierce response. Much classical viral disease, e.g. serum hepatitis (hepatitis B) is in fact due to destruction of the infected liver cells by a host reaction. If such destruction were to persist at a less intense level and affect organs not apparently massively infected by virus, it would be classified as auto-immune. It thus becomes a fine point whether the disease is primarily viral or auto-immune, the virus being the cause and the auto-antibodies the pathogenic mechanism.

The normal defence against this catastrophe is the total elimination of the virus by antibody and complement (p. 32). The defence may fail and virus persist if complement is qualitatively or quantitatively deficient. Under such circumstances the antibody merely removes viral antigen from the cell surface and thereby renders the virus immune to attack. This in turn leads to viral persistence and possibly to the unpleasant auto-immune sequelae described above. There is a strong association of particular HLA sub-types (p. 220) with auto-immune diseases. In some cases the link may be the increased liability of certain HLA genes to permit viral persistance.

Bibliography *(Chapters 6, 7, 8, 9)*

Amos D B, Schwartz R S, Janicki B W (eds) 1979 Immune Mechanisms and Disease. Academic Press, New York.

Cohen S, Ward P A, McCluskey R T (eds) 1979 Mechanisms of Immunopathology. Wiley, New York

Roitt, I 1977 Essential Immunology. 3rd edn. Blackwell, Oxford

Turk J L 1978 Immunology in clinical medicine 3rd edn. Heinemann, London

Weir D M 1977 Immunology: an outline for students of medicine and biology. 4th edn. Churchill Livingstone, Edinburgh

10

Inflammation

Invertebrates, with no true circulatory system, respond to an irritant by surrounding it with specialised cells (haematocytes) which then ingest it. If the damage is very severe the invertebrate simply rejects the injured portion of its anatomy as a prelude to its regeneration. In higher forms of life, including man, the local reaction to injury is much more complex because of the evolution of the circulatory system, and disappearance of the kind of major regenerative powers possessed by the earthworm. This local reaction to injury is called inflammation, from the Latin word *inflamare*, meaning to burn. The name is apt because when the skin reacts in this way, it is red, hot, swollen and tender (the four cardinal signs of inflammation described by Celsus in AD 35). Inflammation also causes loss of function as first pointed out by Virchow and stressed by John Hunter with the common sense of the practical surgeon.

Although any tissues may suffer injury, inflammation is essentially the reaction to injury of the living microcirculation and its contents. Inflammation of an organ is commonly designated by adding the suffix – itis, as in appendicitis. Injury is most commonly bacterial infection, i.e. a breakdown of symbiosis such as to produce demonstrable tissue damage. However, excessive heat or cold, irritant chemicals or trauma or antigen/antibody reactions can lead to similar results. The microcirculation (that part which can be seen only with the aid of the light microscope) includes arterioles, venules, capillaries and lymphatics. Its contents comprise the fluid and cellular constituents of the blood (Fig. 10.1). Inflammation may be acute, ie. of short duration or chronic, i.e. prolonged, depending on the nature of the injury, and both have their characteristic pattern although in chronic inflammation there are usually preliminary and sometimes recurrent acute phases.

Acute inflammation
The changes in the small blood vessels which constitute an acute inflammatory reaction can be seen in transparent structures such as

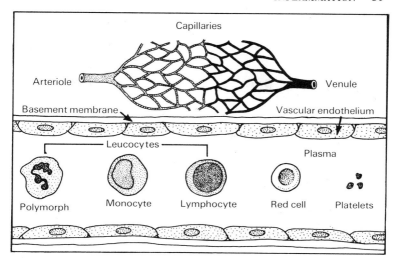

Fig. 10.1 The microcirculation and its contents.

the web of the frog's foot or by inserting a transparent perspex disc into the rabbit's ear. The reaction is essentially a stereotyped sequence of events. Immediately after entry of the irritant stimulus there is a brief constriction of arterioles followed by their prolonged dilatation. This leads to flushing of the capillary network with blood and the opening up of dormant capillary channels. There is also dilatation of venules and lymphatics (Fig. 10.2). The blood flow is increased and may remain so or may become sluggish. The white cells of the blood,

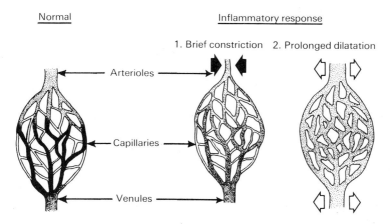

Fig. 10.2 The response of the microcirculation to local injury.

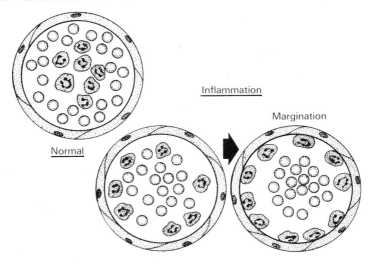

Fig. 10.3 Margination of leucocytes in acute inflammation

the leucocytes, leave the centre of the stream which they normally occupy to move to the periphery. They then form a layer against the inner surface of the cells which line the lumen of the blood vessels, the vascular endothelium, a process known as margination and which is a prelude to the migration of leucocytes through the vessel wall into the adjacent tissues (Fig. 10.3).

At the same time a crucial change occurs in the wall of the venules and capillaries. These vessels are normally freely permeable to water and small solutes but only slightly permeable to plasma proteins, i.e. albumin, the globulins and fibrinogen. In fact, it is the oncotic pressure of these retained molecules which counters the hydrostatic pressure of the blood. This oncotic pressure keeps water inside the vessels whereas the tangential thrust of the blood pressure pushes it out through the vessel wall like a positive pressure filter. In inflammation, hydrostatic pressure inside the vessel may rise, the balance be upset and more water may leave the blood and enter the tissues. More important, the wall of the venule and capillary now loses its impermeability to protein. As a result, albumin, globulins and fibrinogen pour out through the wall into the tissues, which thus come to contain fluid with a composition similar to that of blood plasma (Fig. 10.4). The swelling of the tissues is known as oedema and the fluid itself is the fluid exudate. The change in the properties of the vessel wall is called increased vascular permeability. It is demonstrated not only by the high plasma protein levels in the inflammatory oedema but also by observing experimentally the passage through the vessel wall of plasma albumin linked to a coloured azo dye such as trypan blue. Another experimental method is to introduce into the circulation a visible colloid, usually carbon, with a particle size comparable to molecules of plasma protein. The carbon can be seen lying within and outside the walls of permeable vessels especially if instead of making ordinary sections, the tissue is rendered translucent with a clearing agent such as glycerine, spead out and examined under a low power microscope.

The protein which collects outside the vessels is gradually removed by way of the lymphatics. Since the proteins include immunoglobulins and complement, it is obvious that their presence will accelerate the destruction of any bacteria in the vicinity (p. 29). The fibrinogen in the exudate is converted to insoluble fibrin by the usual process of blood coagulation in which a terminal peptide is split off by a ubiquitous and readily activated protease called thrombin, the residue then polymerising. Pathologists have long pondered over whether fibrin in exudates is of any value to the host, e.g. by acting as a mechanical barrier to the spread of bacteria. Although fibrin is a very prominent feature of many inflammatory exudates, its benefit to the host in these circumstances is still in doubt although in the control of bleeding it is essential for life itself (p. 141). Whether or not fibrin hampers bacterial spread its effects in inflammation can be harmful to the host. It leads to knitting

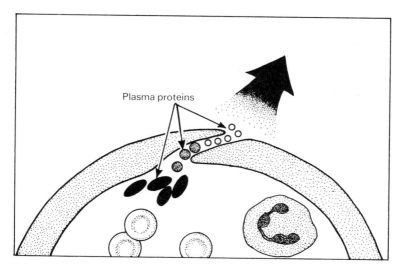

Fig. 10.4 Increased permeability of venule to plasma proteins. The proteins escape in inverse proportion to the molecular size (molecular sieving).

together of previously free surfaces such as the pericardium, with impairment of function and in diphtheria, where it forms a dense membrane in the throat, it frequently caused death by asphyxiation. For good or ill, however, its presence in exudates is simply a consequence of leakage of fibrinogen through permeable vessels and its inevitable subsequent conversion to fibrin.

It is plain that increased vascular permeability to protein causes great discomfort both to invading micro-organisms and to the host. It tends to develop in a complex multiphasic way depending on the nature and severity of injury. It may last for less than an hour or for several days, perhaps weeks, with leakage from both venules and capillaries. The electron microscope has shown that the protein escapes through gaps which appear between endothelial cells in the vessel wall, replacing the tight oblique intercellular junctions of the normal vessel. These newly formed channels are the escape route even in fenestrated vessels which as in the gut exhibit permanent discontinuities between endothelium. Similarly, the intracytoplasmic transport pathway which exists in endothelial cells appears to be almost entirely ignored in inflammation. Most of these facts have been established by the use of small marker molecules such as carbon or ferritin and this technique shows such particles and presumably plasma protein to be temporarily detained by the vascular basement membrane. Plasma proteins leave these leaky vessels with an ease roughly proportional to their concentration in the blood and inversely proportional to the size of their molecule (molecular sieving). Selective escape of plasma proteins could therefore result from gel-filtration through the basement membrane or it could be due to differential concentration-dependent rates of bulk flow. A major cause of the inter-endothelial gaps is active contraction of the endothelial cells due to the action of chemical mediators such as histamine. Only the endothelial cells of venules are affected; capillaries seem not to respond to these mediators, although they leak plasma protein after direct injury. In their response to mediators, venular endothelium behave like smooth muscle. As they contract they shrink away from each other thus allowing channels to form between them (Fig. 10.5). The contraction is accomplished by the intracytoplasmic network of microtubules and fibrils and involves the contractile protein actomyosin and the utilisation of energy. It is likely that the widely distributed substance, cyclic AMP, together with the enzyme which forms it, adenyl cyclase, regulates this process. In many types of injury e.g. burns, significant leakage occurs as a result of structural disruption of the vessel wall. Such change affects both capillaries and venules. Direct damage of this sort also causes these vessels to leak by loosening the inter-endothelial junctions, a kind of unzipping effect. In summary, increased vascular permeability can be due both to direct ethothelial damage affecting capillaries and venules, and to the action of chemical mediators causing endothelial contraction only in venules.

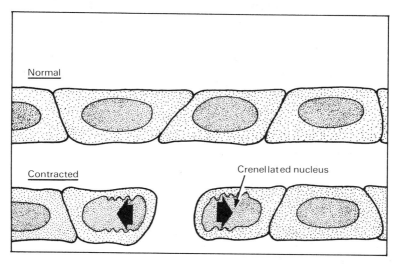

Fig. 10.5 Contraction of vascular endothelium to allow escape of plasma protein.

To qualify for the title of mediator of inflammation a substance should reproduce some or all of the inflammatory changes in low concentration, be demonstrable at the inflamed site at the appropriate time and inhibition of the substance, e.g. by drugs, should lead to suppression of some or all of the inflammatory phenomena. Needless to say, these criteria are seldom fulfilled completely. One of the best documented mediators is histamine, which is widely distributed in body tissues and formed by histidine decarboxylase from the amino acid histidine. Histamine is released by all kinds of local injury and some of it comes from degranulated mast cells. In very mild transient inflammation, e.g. the 'triple response' (flare, erythema and wheal) described by Lewis and provoked by firm stroking of the skin, histamine together with a vasodilator axon reflex probably accounts for all the changes and in other examples, e.g. vasomotor rhinitis (hay fever) accounts for the majority. In more severe inflammation, histamine is responsible only for the earliest changes, seen in the initial half hour or so. Another amine, 5-hydroxytryptamine (Serotonin, 5-HT) not found in human mast cells but present in platelets, may also be important at this stage. Local inactivation of adrenalin or noradrenalin

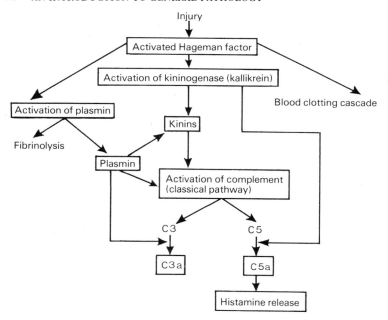

Fig. 10.6 The interaction of Hageman Factor, proteases, kinins, complement, blood clotting, fibrinolysis and histamine release following local injury.

may also play a role, since the effect of these substances, if unopposed would be to inhibit the inflammatory response.

It seems likely that mediators operate in sequence and that after the phase of histamine and 5-HT release and adrenalin inactivation, vascular changes are kept going by activation of the kinin system (Fig. 10.6). Kinins are polypeptides composed of 8—10 amino acids. They are present in blood as inactive precursors, kininogens, converted to the active form by widely distributed plasma and tissue enzymes (kininogenases) and then rapidly inactivated by other enzymes called kininases. Activation is a complex process which shares some of the factors in the cascade pathway involved in blood clotting. More specifically, initiation of the kinin cascade occurs as a result of contact of Hageman factor (Clotting factor XII) with negatively charged surfaces. These surfaces include the ubiquitous collagen, so activation is easily achieved. The evidence for the participation of kinins in inflammation is somewhat tenuous since they are elusive substances, but depletion of bodily stores of the precursor by injection of cellulose sulphate does diminish the post-histamine phase of inflammatory oedema. The role of histamine is easily demonstrated by giving doses of anti-histamine drugs which specifically antagonise the substance or by depleting the body of its stores of histamine by injecting histamine releasers. Only H1 histamine receptors seem to be involved in inflammation. Drugs which block H2 receptors and therefore interfere with histamine-mediated gastric secretion have no effect on the inflammatory process.

Although the kinins have a probable role, albeit ill-defined, as inflammatory mediators, recent attention has been more directed to the ubiquitous family of prostaglandins and thromboxanes. This family consists of long chain compounds composed of polyunsaturated fatty acids (Fig 10.7). All are formed in or on cells from arachidonic acid by cyclo-oxygenase and have numerous pharmacological actions. Indeed, some prostaglandins have effects directly opposed to those of other prostaglandins. Thus some increase vascular permeability and others diminish it. Another important effect of prostaglandins is to potentiate the actions of histamine and kinins in increasing vascular permeability. It may be that prostaglandins situated as they are on cell surfaces, especially on mobile leucocytes, represent a widely distributed and

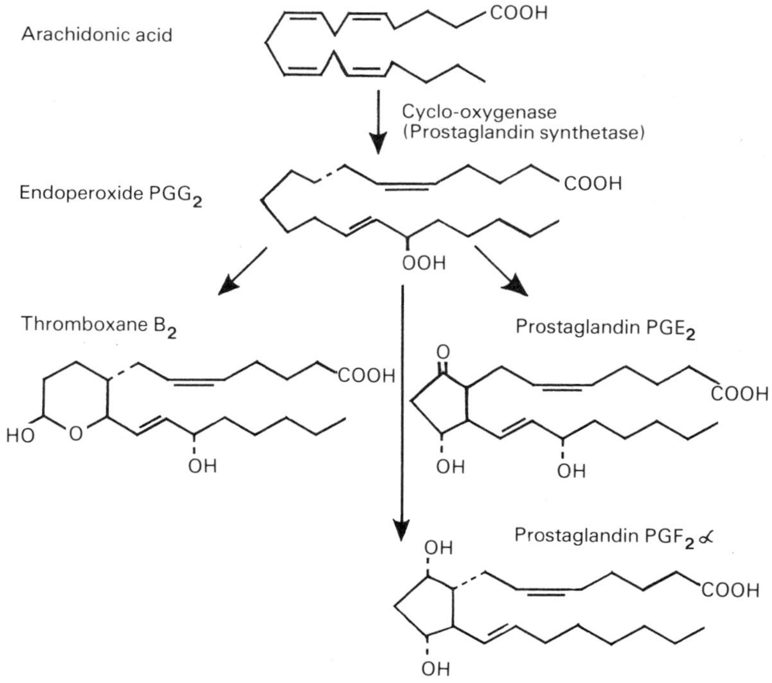

Fig. 10.7 The formation of endoperoxides, thromboxanes and prostaglandins from arachidonic acid.

self-contained regulatory system able to initiate, maintain or suppress inflammation according to circumstances. These opposing effects are probably achieved by way of the cyclic AMP/adenyl cyclase system. An excess of cyclic AMP restrains the contractility and mobility of cells possibly by stimulating the phosphorylation of the protein of the intracellular micro-tubules and fibrils. It could be predicted that prostaglandins with opposite biological effects would have opposite actions on the cyclic AMP/adenyl cyclase system.

Slow reacting substance (SRS) is a lipid mediator which increases vascular permeability but which may be particularly important in causing bronchial constriction in asthma (p. 42). It is released from cells and is probably a member of the prostaglandin family.

The sequential appearance of mediators each dependent on a complex cascade of enzyme reactions (Fig. 10.8), seems an absurdly complicated way of dilating vessels and making them leak. However, bearing in mind the unvarying nature of the acute inflammatory response, even in widely different species, and the enormous variety of eliciting stimuli, the intervention of a final common pathway between injury and reaction seems a likely mechanism to have evolved.

A mediator of importance, not yet discussed, is complement. Two peptides derived from the 3rd or 5th components, known as C3a and C5a respectively, cause inflammatory oedema when injected locally, e.g. into skin. They do so partly by direct action and partly by liberation from mast cells of histamine. This latter action is known as

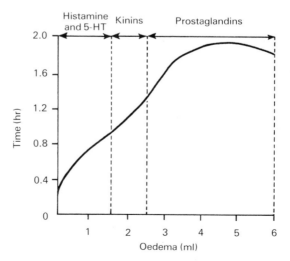

Fig. 10.8 Sequential release of mediators of increased vascular permeability.

the anaphylotoxin effect. It is becoming clear that C5a is the most powerful mediator of the two. For C3a and C5a to be released it is first necessary for the complement cascade to be activated by the classical or alternate pathway (p. 28). C3 and C5 are then split by a variety of blood and tissue enzymes.

The complement system interacts closely with another mediator of acute inflammation, the kinin system. The inter-relationship is shown in Figure 10.6. The figure shows the key role of the Hageman factor in activating both systems via the proteases plasmin and kallikrein. The additional links with blood clotting on the one hand and fibrinolysis on the other, are not unexpected since all these systems are essentially homeostatic in the face of injury and could be predicted to evolve together.

Other mediators of the vascular events of acute inflammation have been canvassed. These include a wide range of lysosomal enzymes and cationic proteins and of lymphokines (p. 34). In general however, the substance acting on the microcirculation is either an amine (e.g. histamine), a peptide (e.g. kinins, complement fragments) or an acidic lipid (e.g. prostaglandins).

Although the importance of antibodies and phagocytosis in destroying bacteria is obvious, the survival value of the vascular changes *per se* could be disputed. It has, however, been shown that small inoculations of bacteria which are killed within a few minutes before any phagocytes arrive at the area, survive and multiply if the early dilatation and

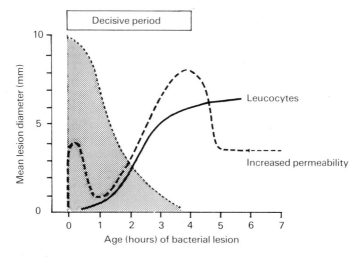

Fig. 10.9 Relationship of killing of small inoculations of bacteria to inflammatory response (Based on the work of A.A. Miles and colleagues).

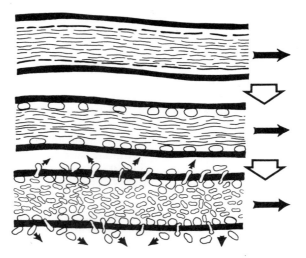

Fig. 10.10 Margination and migration of leucocytes.

increased permeability of vessels is prevented by injection of adrenalin (Fig. 10.9). In other instances, e.g. in lobar pneumonia, the inflammatory oedema probably facilitates spread of the bacteria and may lead to death of the host. In other words increased vascular flow and permeability bring antibody and other bactericidal agents to the scene but also accelerate the spread of those germs which survive. Similarly, increased lymph flow carries bacteria to the local lymph nodes which are well adapted for bacterial killing but which are also key junctions in any spread throughout the body.

Increased blood flow, access of plasma proteins to extra-vascular tissues and mobilisation of phagocytes are the features of acute inflammation which have survival value for the host. It would be expected therefore that the exudation of fluid would rapidly be augmented by the arrival of phagocytes (Fig. 10.10). Indeed, within half an hour of injury, leucocytes are seen to migrate from the blood into the tissues, doing so by inserting pseudopodia into the inter-endothelial junctions and then wriggling through the vessel wall by amoeboid motion, somehow getting across the basement membrane without obviously destroying it (Fig. 10.11). At this stage the leucocytes involved are neutrophil granulocytes but they may shortly be joined by monocytes. Red cells and platelets also pass out of the vessel in the wake of the leucocytes or via inter-endothelial gaps. The infiltration of these cells, especially the leucocytes is known as the cellular exudate (Fig. 10.12).

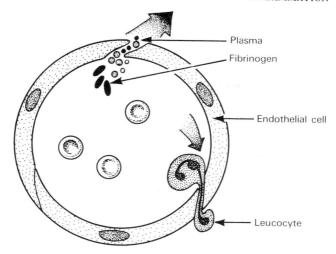

Fig. 10.11 Increased vascular permeability and leucocyte emigration in acute inflammation.

The emigration of white cells requires the leucocytes to expend energy and this demands that they be stimulated in some way. Injury seldom directly persuades leucocytes to adhere to vessels and migrate through their walls. This important effect is achieved by activation of a further group of chemical mediators. In theory leucocyte emigration could be brought about simply by an acceleration of the natural random amoeboid movement of the cells or by true chemotaxis i.e. direct attraction to a chemical target at the area of damage.

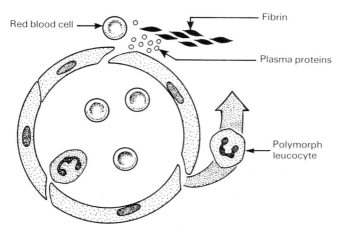

Fig. 10.12 The acute inflammatory exudate.

The response of leucocytes is most easily studied outside the body in a device called the Boyden Chamber. In this the leucocytes are suspended in fluid on top of a filter containing pores of from 3—8 μm in diameter. Below the filter is another chamber containing the fluid whose chemotactic powers are under test. If the substances cause leucocyte migration the cells will fight their way through the small pores and accumulate on the under surface of the filter disc. If the active substance is in the bottom chamber only, the cells will show increased mobility and also migrate in that direction, indicating chemotaxis. If the active substance is on both sides of the filter the leucocytes will show enhanced mobility but no particular tendency to move across the filter, exhibiting accelerated random movement only. If the active substance is confined to the top chamber with the cells, the leucocytes will exhibit increased mobility but will not leave the chamber in significant numbers, indicating a localising effect (Fig. 10.13). Although there is some difference of opinion, these experiments seem to show that substances which attract leucocytes may cause true chemotaxis, accelerated random movement or trapping depending on whether the concentration gradient of the substance relative to the leucocyte is positive, non-existent or negative. All three situations probably exist in different zones of an inflamed area and are conducive to leucocyte accumulation in acute inflammation.

Many substances cause leucocytes to show chemotaxis and increased movement. With a few exceptions, however, they all require the presence of fresh serum before they can exert their effect. The main obligatory factor in serum, although probably not the only one, is complement which as we have learned (p. 28) is a complex assortment

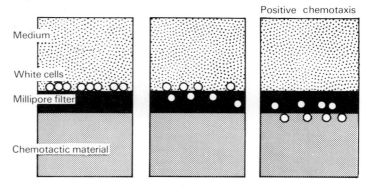

Fig. 10.13 The demonstration of leucocyte chemotaxis in the Boyden chamber.

of plasma proteins, constituting a cascade of enzyme reactions and playing an important role in the removal of bacteria. When suitably activated, complement generates peptides known as C3a and C5a which are chemotactic for white cells and which are split off from the third (C3) and fifth component (C5). Biological material which forms these chemotactic molecules from complement includes many and possibly all bacterial species, fungi, antigen/antibody complexes, tissue breakdown products, granules (lysosomes) from leucocytes and bacterial endotoxin. The mode of action of C3 and C5 products on leucocytes is not known but enhanced mobility is almost certainly due to activity of the cytoplasmic microtubules involving the cooperation of cyclic AMP on the cell surface. It is possible that prostaglandins also on the cell surface are involved, as well as esterase enzymes in the leucocyte membrane (Fig. 10.14).

With the possible exception of prostaglandins, no inflammatory mediators other than complement fragments are chemotactic for leucocytes. Of the complement fragments, those derived from C5 seem to be most potent.

The pattern of leucocyte infiltration varies with the nature and age of the inflammatory lesion. Neutrophil granulocytes are usually replaced progressively by monocytes with the passage of time and in some types of damage, due for example to helminths or Type I hypersensitivity, eosinophil granulocytes predominate. Monocyte predominance could be due simply to disappearance of the more short lived granulocytes since both cell types usually emigrate concurrently.

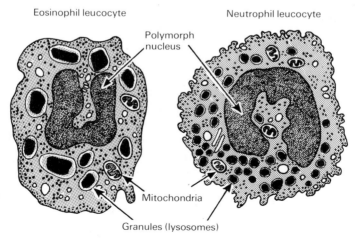

Fig. 10.14 Drawing of the electron microscopic appearances of a neutrophil and an eosinophil leucocyte.

It is probable, however, that complement or other serum factors generate substances which are more chemotactic for one type of leucocyte than another.

Such semi-specific factors have been identified for neutrophils, eosinophils, monocytes and even for B lymphocytes, although the ability of lymphocytes, to respond to chemotaxis is not universally accepted.

The adhesion of leucocytes to the luminal surface of vascular endothelium prior to their emigration has produced many hypothetical explanations such as reduction in negative charge at the surfaces (to overcome mutual repulsion) or the secretion of some adhesive chemical. It seems quite likely, however, that the apparently adherent leucocyte is merely in the initial stage of migration and of response to a chemotactic substance which may have become adsorbed to the inner surface of the vascular wall.

Suppuration
The life of a neutrophil granulocyte is measured in days and they seldom, if ever, survive the act of ingesting and killing micro-organisms. It is possible that the metabolic activity of destroying and dissolving the organisms (p. 18) hastens the death of the cells. In other cases it is obvious that the bacteria are more effective at killing the leucocyte than vice versa and if untreated by antibiotics this will lead eventually to the death of the patient. Suppuration is an intermediate situation with two main components. Very large numbers of granulocytes are summoned into the tissues usually by the chemotactic influence of certain bacteria notably the *Staphylococcus aureus*. The exuded leucocytes are killed in large numbers by the bacteria and their bodies liquefied by their own lysosomal enzymes to form a creamy viscous fluid rich in lipids, proteins and nucleic acids and known as pus. The mass of bacteria, dead, dying and liquefied leucocytes and surviving inflamed tissue is termed an abscess. When present in skin as it commonly is it is called a boil or if very large, a carbuncle. The painful abscess is the price we pay for survival since it is an inevitable result of confining certain dangerous bacteria to one part of the body rather than allowing them to disseminate.

Inflammation and the nervous system
Many experiments have shown that inflammation proceeds unmodified in the absence of any nerve supply. This does not mean, however, that the nervous system is unable to influence the inflammatory reaction. At the simplest level, the red flare that surrounds the skin reaction to mild trauma (the triple response) is abolished if the sensory

or vasomotor nerves are blocked or cut. In a more complex situation, hypnosis can persuade a subject with exactly similar areas of mild damage on each of his arms that one will produce an inflammatory reaction and the other not and that one arm is painful and the other not. Interestingly, only the vascular changes are affected by hypnotic suggestion, leucocyte migration proceeding equally in the two arms.

The converse situation, where suggestion causes an inflammatory reaction to appear, is commonplace in patients with Type I hypersensitivity (p. 43). In these patients emotional factors may determine whether contact with the sensitising antigen will or will not induce increased vascular permeability in the nose, eyes or skin.

Emotion may possibly influence the onset or severity of inflammation in more serious diseases such as ulcerative colitis. All diseases in which emotional factors seem likely to play a major role are known as psychosomatic, but they should not be confused with unhappiness *per se* which may produce symptoms of organic disease without the physical stigmata (p. 275).

Generally speaking, emotion and suggestion affect only those pathological phenomena readily influenced by the autonomic nervous system. Thus vascular permeability may be restrained by neurogenic adrenalin release and result in vasoconstriction, or be exaggerated by depression of those same forces, whereas leucocyte emigration could not be reached by them. Enthusiasm for the role of psychic factors in inflammatory diseases, such as ulcerative colitis or peptic ulcer, has waned somewhat. The consensus view at the moment is that tangible agents cause these conditions but that the patient's emotional state may raise or lower the level of the inflammatory response to them.

Pain

The heat, redness and swelling of acute inflammation are explained by vascular dilatation and increased vascular permeability. The pain is due partly to pressure on sensory nerve endings by the exuded fluid, especially if the space in which it can expand is limited (Fig. 10.15) and partly to the release of bodily substances which stimulate these nerves. In fact all the chemical mediators which are responsible for the vascular changes also cause pain. These are histamine, serotonin, kinins and prostaglandins, kinins being particularly effective while histamine release may lead merely to itching, as in urticaria. Prostaglandins may act by lowering the threshold of response to other pain-producing substances. Other chemicals liberated by nervous stimuli or cell injury, e.g. acetylcholine or potassium ions may also be painful.

The survival value to the host of pain is obvious since it tells him that

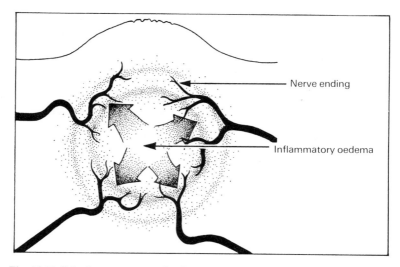

Fig. 10.15 Pain due to pressure of inflammatory exudate on nerve ending.

the injured part must be favoured and rested and that appropriate action, especially retreat, should be considered. The reverse side of the coin is represented by the disability caused by pain itself.

In the context of survival it is important to realise that although pain is invoked by stimulation of sensory nerve endings its appreciation is dependent on subjective factors. Soldiers receiving wounds in battle that would normally produce incapacitating pain will ignore the injury and even refuse morphia if by doing so their chances of survival are improved by remaining mobile and alert. Only when safety is reached will they experience real pain. Comparable wounds received in civilian life, e.g. in traffic accidents, will be experienced as severe pain almost immediately. These observations show that the sensation of pain is determined ultimately in the higher centres of the brain and that it can be overridden by more urgent survival mechanisms such as the need for flight or self defence. Since crippling wounds can be rendered painless by this expression of the brain's higher centres it should not surprise us that hypnosis or autosuggestion should have a similar power over more trivial injuries.

The discovery of the endorphins, endogenous pain-suppressing opiates produced in the brain, pituitary and adrenal and acting on the cerebrum, provide a pharmacological basis for these variations in the perception of pain. They also offer a possible explanation for the impressive local anaesthesia sometimes achieved by acupuncture, if as some believe, appropriate insertion of needles generates release of endorphins.

Bibliography

Majno B, Palade G E 1961 Studies on inflammation I & II. Journal of Biophysical and Biochemical Cytology (now Journal of Cell Biology) II: 571-607

Ryan G B, Majno G 1977 Acute inflammation. American Journal of Pathology 86: 185

Sorkin E (ed) 1974 Chemotaxis: its biology and biochemistry. Karger, Basel

Weissmann G, Samuelsson B, Paoletti R (eds) 1979 Advances in inflammation research. vol 1, Raven Press, New York

Willoughy D A, Giroud J P, Velo G P 1977 Perspectives in inflammation. MTP, Lancaster

Zweifach B W, Grant L, McCluskey R T (eds) 1974 The inflammatory process. 2nd edn. vols 1, 2, 3. Academic Press, New York

11

Healing and repair

Taking living organisms in general, the basic response to destruction or loss of tissues insufficient to cause death, is to regenerate and reconstitute the part which has gone. This law operates all the way up to the lower vertebrates and the salamander will replace an amputated limb as readily and as faithfully as the earthworm its body segments. It is often stated that mammals have lost their regenerative capacity but as a generalisation this is only partially true. If a hole is punched right through a rabbit's ear all the tissues which have gone will be replaced including cartilage, skin, hair and glands. However, in no other mammal studied does the ear have this capacity. On the other hand even in man some organs can regenerate as satisfactorily as the salamander's limb. Another frequent generalisation is that the more differentiated or specialised a tissue the less its capacity to grow again. This pronouncement probably derives from the observation that brain cells, admittedly highly specialised, never regenerate whereas simpler mesenchynal cells divide readily. Between these extremes, however, there are so many exceptions that the general statement becomes invalid. Liver cells are certainly highly differentiated and with many specialised functions but regenerate as fast as any other human tissue. Muscle cells which are specialised only in being contractile, regenerate poorly. Lung tissue, which is fairly simple, is reluctant to grow again in adult life. Kidney tubule cells, less specialised than liver epithelium, regenerate poorly. There must be reasons for these discrepancies but they remain unknown and do not conform to any general law or pattern yet apparent.

It is important to clarify the relationship between wounding, healing and regeneration. A wound implies structural damage with loss of tissue and most commonly refers to local destruction of the integument, i.e. the skin. Similarly, healing can refer to the restoration of any part but is most commonly used in relation to the body surface so that wound healing generally implies reconstitution of the integrity of the skin. The major exception to this statement in human disease is the healing infarct (p. 150) especially of the cardiac muscle. In a cardiac infarct many muscle cells die but lack regenerative powers. However, there is an inflammatory reaction and the exudate and dead muscle cells become replaced by connective tissue and eventually converted to a dense scar by the process described in the next few pages.

In theory regeneration could occur independently of wound healing but in practice this is hardly ever the case. Where it appears to do so special factors operate, e.g. in the lens of the salamander eye where the new lens is formed from the adjacent iris. Most other examples are really instances of organ hyperplasia (p. 191) due to increased stimulation, e.g. by hormones. On the other hand experiments have made it clear that classical regeneration, as in the growth of new limbs in newts or salamanders after amputation depends upon healing of the overlying skin wound. If healing is prevented, e.g. by covering the stump with old skin which will not 'take', the limb does not regenerate. The stimulus for the complex regrowth of the mesenchymal structures of the limb appears to come from the piled up epithelial cap of the healing skin provided that it is reached by an adequate nerve supply. Degree of innervation seems to be crucial and there have been several successes in inducing partial regeneration of amputated limbs in frogs, lizards and newborn opossums by augmenting the local nerve supply. In mammals, cyclical regrowth of male deer antlers after they are shed, offers another example of complex regeneration and restoration of architecture being dependent on healing of the associated wound of the integument.

It is necessary to clarify these relationships because healing as it occurs in man is sometimes thought of wrongly as a somewhat inadequate substitute for genuine regeneration. In fact healing is both a prerequisite for regeneration of other tissues and a form of regeneration in its own right, in which there is regrowth of covering epithelium and underlying connective tissue.

The similarity between regeneration and wound healing is brought out by the historical fact that the events of healing were first observed by the microscope in living tissues in the amputated stump of the tadpoles tail and subsequently confirmed by the device of inserting a transplant chamber into a wound made in the rabbit's ear. Wound healing implies three processes; the regeneration of tissues that have been destroyed, e.g. the reconstitution of skin epithelium, the regeneration of damaged connective tissue and the replacement by fibrous tissue of dead cells which cannot regenerate. The healing process as a whole is best thought of in the same way as acute inflammation, i.e. as a consistent sequence of events.

When a wound occurs there is rupture of blood vessels with escape

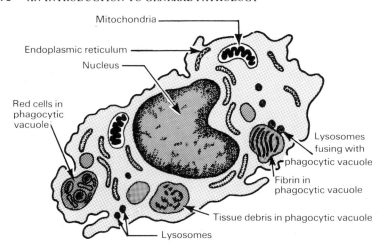

Fig. 11.1 Drawing of the electron microscopic appearance of a macrophage after phagocytosis of fibrin, red cells and tissue debris.

of blood. If the body made no provision for this contingency the patient would bleed to death. Fortunately there are efficient mechanisms for stopping the bleeding within minutes (p. 140) but the wounded tissues fill up with partially solidified blood before haemostasis, as the control of bleeding is known, is complete. The original tissue damage plus the presence of so much extravascular blood, is sufficient to initiate inflammatory changes in the adjacent intact blood vessels and there is a migration of leucocytes into the wound area. The stimulus for polymorph attraction is short-lived, as are the polymorphs themselves, so their appearance is fleeting. More important is the emigration of monocytes, possibly directed by local formation of chemotactic factors semi-specific for these cells. Once in the tissues, monocytes mature into macrophages, active phagocytes capable of ingesting and digesting large amounts of debris (Fig. 11.1). Macrophages are probably essential for wound healing since their destruction by the deliberate injection of antibodies directed specifically against them seems to interfere with repair quite substantially. Similar removal of polymorphs, however, does not affect wound healing.

The accummulation of macrophages and the digestion of debris is the first requisite for repair of connective tissue and takes several days. Within a week, however, there are clear signs that new blood vessels are growing into the wounded area (Fig. 11.2). These appear first as solid cords of endothelial cells growing out as buds from the surviving capillaries at the wound edge (Fig. 11.3). The cells arise by mitotic

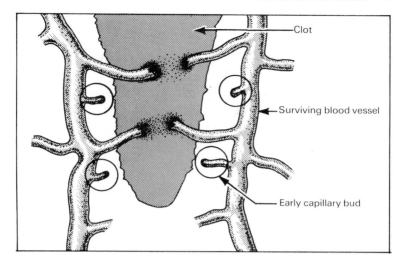

Fig. 11.2 Ingrowth of capillary buds in wound.

activity in the endothelial cells of the parent vessel followed by their migration in the direction of the wound. The endothelial buds grow at about 0.1—0.6 mm per day and if the macrophages have not done their work properly and the clot is too solid their progress may be severely restricted. Mitotic division occurs also in the endothelium of the bud itself about 0.5 mm from its tip and there is a strong tendency for buds

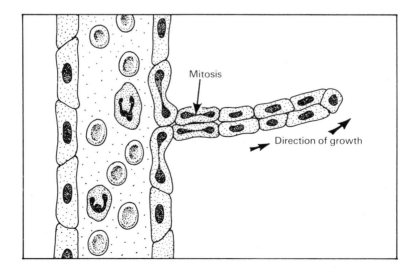

Fig. 11.3 Ingrowth of solid bud of endothelium.

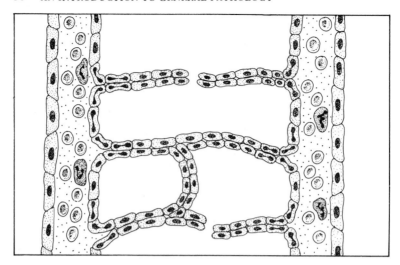

Fig. 11.4 Ingrowth of regenerating blood vessels to form arcades and loops

to join with each other to form loops or arcades (Fig. 11.4). The solid endothelial cords become canalised within hours and in the lumen so formed blood begins to flow (Fig. 11.5). The young vessels are leaky and are surrounded by plasma, red corpuscles and leucocytes that have escaped (Fig. 11.5) but they provide the second essential prerequisite for regeneration of connective tissue, i.e. a blood supply. At first all the

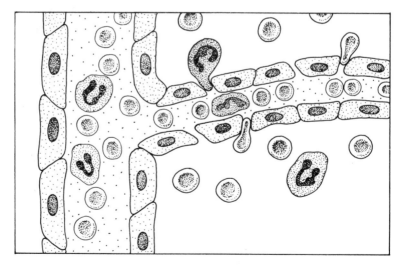

Fig. 11.5 New capillary bud develops a lumen.

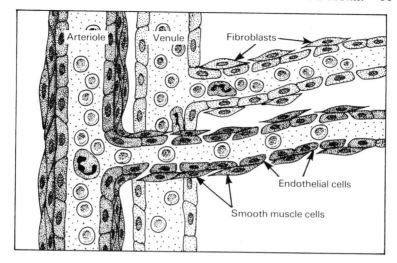

Fig. 11.6 Transformation of new vessels into arterioles and venules.

vessels are simple capillaries but soon some differentiate into arterioles and venules, in the former case by acquiring a coat of smooth muscle cells (Fig. 11.6). Newly formed arterioles acquire a vasomotor nerve supply sometimes as early as two weeks after wounding.

Soon an extensive remodelling process occurs, many of the original capillary loops disappearing by a kind of shrivelling of redundant vessels, so that the blood supply to the wound becomes gradually reduced. In parallel with the ingrowth of blood vessels, but quite separately, the lymphatic circulation becomes re-established by a similar sequence of budding and joining. Lymphatic endothelium appears to have an unerring instinct for joining other lymphatic loops but avoiding blood channels.

Vasomotor nerves have already been mentioned but other sensory and motor nerves also regenerate but more slowly. This occurs by the formation of sprouts which grow from the central portion of the cut end pushing through a guide channel formed by proliferating sheath (Schwann) cells and acquiring a myelin sheath in the process (Fig. 11.7). The nerves grow at about 0.2–0.4 mm each day.

Any regenerating tissue must obviously develop new blood vessels, lymphatics and nerves. The special feature of reconstituted connective tissue is fibroblast activity. The fibroblast is the basic mesenchymal cell of adult tissue whose main property is the synthesis of the constituents of connective tissue, namely collagen and mucopolysaccharides (Fig. 11.8). The osteoblast and chondrocyte which form bone and cartilage

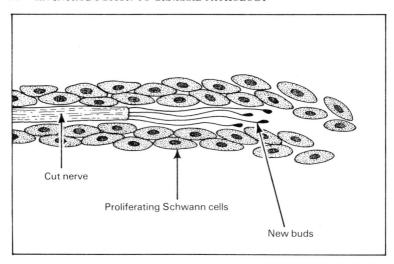

Fig. 11.7 Regeneration of damaged nerve.

respectively, are its close cousins. The fibroblast is an elongated cell distinguished mainly by an impressive maze of rough endoplasmic reticulum lining wide cisternae in its cytoplasm. Closely related to the exterior of the cell, the electron microscope commonly reveals bundles of collagen with their characteristic regular transverse banding. The fibroblast appears so promptly and in such large numbers in healing wounds that there has been much speculation as to its origin. In

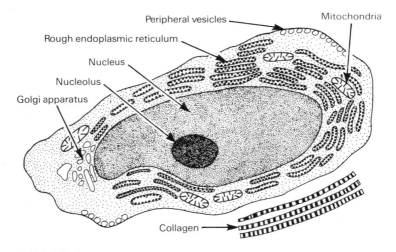

Fig. 11.8 Fibroblast.

particular, pathologists have been attracted to the idea that these fibroblasts are derived from the monocytes or lymphocytes found in the wound at an earlier stage of healing. It is therefore worthwhile to quote an experiment by Ross, Everett and Tyler which proves this notion to be incorrect. Two rats were joined in parabiotic union, like "Siamese twins", so that their circulation mingled by way of a flap of skin and subcutaneous tissue. This pedicle was then clamped so that no blood could pass from one rat to the other. One rat was then given an isotope of a DNA constituent (^{3}H-thymidine) so that many cells of its body became recognisably labelled. Monocytes, lymphocytes and fibroblasts of this rat were therefore distinguishable from those of its Siamese twin. The unlabelled animal then received a small skin wound and the clamp was released so that their circulations mingled and labelled cells poured into the wounded rat. The wound site became filled with labelled polymorphs, monocytes and macrophages but none of the numerous fibroblasts which appeared in the wound were so labelled. From this and other experiments it can be concluded that the fibroblasts come from pre-existing local fibroblasts. Indeed, these cells in the connective tissue at the wound margin show extensive mitotic activity, following which they and their progeny migrate into the wound itself at the same time as the vascular buds and at a speed of about 0.2 mm per day. In the wound they continue to divide and about six days after their arrival the first collagen fibres are recognisable, with their cross striations at intervals of 64 nm.

The way in which fibroblasts make collagen is now better understood than a few years ago. Collagen is a protein which is assembled on the ribosomes within the endoplasmic reticulum in the usual way. At this stage in its production the protein is known as protocollagen. It contains an unusually high number of molecules of proline and also of lysine. These proline and lysine residues now acquire hydroxyl groups to become the amino acids hydroxyproline and hydroxylysine which are characteristic of collagen. The process catalyzed by the enzyme protocollagen proline hydroxylase is a remarkable one, not least because it occurs after all the RNA-dependent transcriptions on which assembly of the collagen molecule depends have been completed. At this stage the hydroxylated collagen is still soluble, has acquired its characteristic form of a triple helix, and is now called procollagen, or tropocollagen. However, connective tissue collagen is insoluble and if it were not, would be as useless as would be its man-made counterparts nylon or terylene if these fabrics dissolved in water. The problem remains of transferring soluble procollagen out of the fibroblast while simultaneously rendering it insoluble. This difficult task is performed by using a mechanism favoured by the body and utilised in the secretion of other proteins and in the formation of fibrin. Procollagen is synthesised with an extra peptide on the end whose presence confers solubility. At the moment of secretion an enzyme, procollagen peptidase cuts off the terminal peptide residue, whereupon the rest of the collagen molecule promptly polymerises to form the typical insoluble, immensely strong, cross-banded fibres.

The other main constituent of connective tissue is the mucopolysaccharide (glucosaminoglycan) matrix and this too is synthesised by the fibroblast, probably via the Golgi apparatus. Its chemical composition depends on the particular type of connective tissue.

With the passage of time there is orientation and remodelling of the new connective tissue which becomes progressively denser, although most healing wounds reach their optimal strength of union within a few weeks unless the tissue loss was very great. The zone of new dense connective tissue is commonly known as a scar.

The fibroblast has another recently discovered property, that of contractility. To be more precise this is a property of the myofibroblast, a cell with the ultrastructural and functional properties of both fibroblasts and smooth muscle cells. The ability of skin wounds to contract in size in the first week or so, as seen in Fig. 11.9, has long been a puzzle and it used to be taught that it was due to contraction of the collagen fibres themselves. It has now been shown that it is the myo-fibroblast which is responsible for this useful reduction in the size of wounds. The cells contract in response to unknown stimuli but certainly by virtue of their cytoplasmic fibrils of actomyosin. As they do so they pull in the margins of the wound and thus reduce the size of the denuded area.

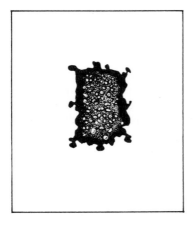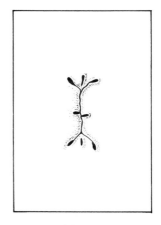

Fig. 11.9 Contraction of a skin wound due to contraction of fibroblasts.

Repair of our body surface has inevitably acquired much emotional charge. If the process were less efficient the subject would no doubt be the source of even more anxiety. The emotive element is revealed in the use of old-fashioned terms such as healing by primary union or first intention, or by secondary union or second intention. Primary union means the healing of a simple incised wound with close apposition of the cut edges. Secondary union means the healing of a wound where there is a substantial tissue defect that has gradually to be filled in and replaced by new connective tissue (Fig. 11.10). Naturally the second type of response takes longer and is more liable to set-backs. This type of healing wound is known also as granulation tissue simply because the regenerating surface looks granular when scrutinised closely. This meaningless term stubbornly remains part of the pathological vocabulary.

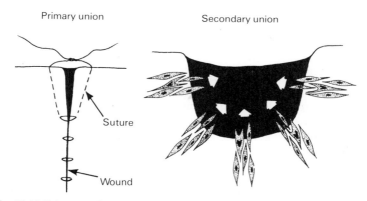

Fig. 11.10 Primary and secondary union.

The events in both types of healing are the same, and under the light microscope one can see all the features described above, the individual picture depending on how far the response has proceeded to completion. Generally a number of young thin-walled blood vessels are visible apparently enmeshed in a pale staining jelly of mucopolysaccharide with variable numbers of fibroblasts, macrophages, granulocytes, red cells and collagen fibrils (Fig. 11.11).

The success of the restoration of the intergrity of skin can be measured by recording the tensile strength of the wound, i.e. the degree of force needed to pull the two edges apart. As little as seven days may be needed to restore tensile strength to normal. The ability to withstand such force is due to the way the polymerised collagen fibres are deposited. Not only do they knit tightly into the adjacent connective

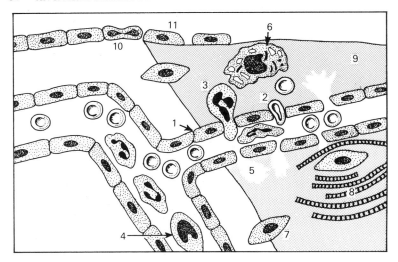

Fig. 11.11 The main features of a healing wound; 1. New vascular endothelium; 2. Dropedesis of red cell; 3. Emigration of leucocyte; 4 Monocyte; 5 Leakage of plasma; 6 Macrophage; 7 Fibroblast; 8 Collagen; 9 Mucopolysaccharide; 10 Proliferating epithelium; 11 Migrating epithelium.

tissue by interweaving of fibres but the strands orientate themselves so as to lie along the lines of maximal stress.

Regeneration of connective tissue is half of wound healing, the other is restoration of the surface epithelium. In skin this is achieved by increased mitotic activity in the epithelium adjacent to the wound margin, especially in the deeper layers. There is also a shortening of the time normally needed to produce daughter cells. The mitotic activity is seen no closer to the wound than 4 or 5 cells, since these 4 or 5 cells have been either damaged or are exposed to unfavourable environmental influences. The stimulus for the onset of mitosis in resting cells and the shortening of the mitotic cycle comes from loss or death of epithelium or from sub-lethal damage to them. Injury to the underlying dermis is not essential for epithelial repair. As proliferation commences, epithelium glide out from the wound margins with a characteristic type of movement quite different from the amoeboid wobble of the migrating leucocyte (Fig. 11.12). The cells use the strands of fibrin in the injured area as guides or conduits in their journey. As the sheets of epithelium from different corners of the wound meet at the centre, the migration and mitosis cease probably as a result of cell-to-cell signals known as contact inhibition. Keratinisation begins quite early. Although hair follicles may contribute daughter epithelium to the newly-formed covering layer it is unusual for hair follicles themselves to regenerate as such and the same is true of sweat

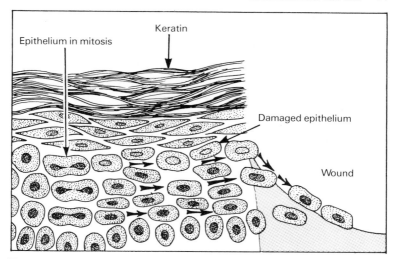

Fig. 11.12 Regenerating surface epithelium dividing and migrating to cover wounded surface.

and sebaceous glands. This is quite likely to be due to local inadequacies, e.g. in nerve supply, rather than to a fundamental deficiency in mammalian development, since as we saw earlier the rabbit's ear has these regenerative powers whereas other parts of the same animal's skin does not.

The prompt and controlled response of epithelium to loss or damage suggests that chemical substances released by injury are organising these events. There is a great deal of uncertainty about this topic and two quite different mechanisms have been advanced as candidates for the role of controller.

The first hypothesis demands that we postulate the existence of a hormone which prevents epithelium from dividing. Compounds which have this effect in living tissues and in organ cultures *in vitro* do exist and are known as chalones (Fig. 11.13). The chalone enthusiasts maintain that after injury chalone action is inhibited and the cells are free to divide until integrity is re-established, upon which chalone effects again dominate. Unfortunately chalones have proved very elusive and after many years of effort have not been consistently characterised although epidermal chalone may be a glycoprotein of 300 000 daltons. It seems possible that they exist, but the verdict is still 'not proven'.

The other mechanism is more substantial in that the active principle has been purified and identified chemically as a peptide of approximately 6000 daltons. This material is the opposite of the chalone in that it actively promotes mitotic division of skin epithelium *in vivo* and in

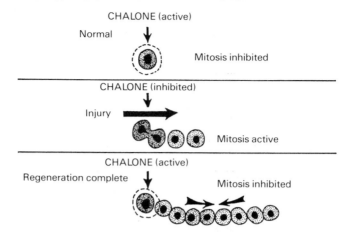

Fig. 11.13 The chalone theory of control of regeneration.

tissue culture. It has the additional properties of promoting keratinisation of epithelium and of accelerating their migration across a surface, both of which would be useful in wound healing. The peptide is known as epidermal growth factor and is normally obtained from the unlikely source of mouse salivary glands (Fig. 11.14). It exists as a precursor complex with protein from which it is released by the enzyme arginine esterase. This could be significant because the same enzyme releases other biologically active peptides, e.g. kinins, relevant to tissue injury. Epidermal growth factor may stimulate mitosis by activating ornithine decarboxylase inside the cell to form polyamines which stimulate synthesis of DNA and RNA.

Regeneration in other organs
Growth factors exist for other types of tissue, e.g. nerves and chalones have been proposed for many varieties of cell. A conspicuous lack of success in identifying chemical controllers exists in the case of the liver. This is disappointing because this organ has remarkable powers of regeneration, in spite of the highly differentiated nature of its constituent cells. The liver's capacity to restore itself is well demonstrated by repeated removal of large portions of the organ from rats. If this is done the liver always reforms to approximately its previous size although not to its precise shape. It has been calculated that in experiments such as these 1 gram of liver generates 18 grams of new liver.

Evidence of mitosis and selective cell death can be found in any normal liver if looked for carefully. After the loss of liver cells by

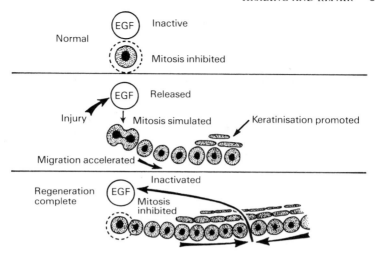

Fig. 11.14 How epidermal growth factor could control regeneration.

surgical extirpation or by chemical or biological damage, the process of liver cell division is greatly augmented. It is this cell proliferation which is responsible for the recovery of organ mass. Most of the mitotic activity takes place at the periphery of the liver lobule but is accompanied by migration of new cells to the centre of the lobule. After partial surgical removal there is also regeneration of the portal tracts including the branches of the portal vein therein as well as hepatic artery radicles and bile ducts. There is preservation of architecture and the newly-formed lobules cannot be distinguished by their microscopic structure from the pre-existing ones.

Well organised regeneration of the liver is of importance in that it demonstrates that this capacity exists in a highly developed organ of mammals and thus dismisses simplistic generalisations about the inverse relationship of differentiation and phylogenetic level on the one hand and re-growth potential on the other. This point is not entirely academic because the artificial stimulation of regeneration could augment transplantation as the answer to organ replacement.

Liver hyperplasia in response to injury also has importance in human pathology because it is a prominent feature of the most important chronic liver disease, i.e. cirrhosis. This is a Greek work referring to the tawny colour (due to iron pigment accumulation) of the afflicted liver. The essential features are a massive overgrowth of the fibrous stroma of the portal tracts, together with proliferation of the bile ducts, coupled with evidence of liver cell death or dysfunction and above all with large areas of liver cell regeneration. The regenerated cells are commonly present in abnormal masses (regeneration nodules) lacking the proper architecture and probably proper function. It seems likely that cirrhosis represents liver regeneration following injury, e.g. due to viruses, malnutrition or alcoholism, in which all the elements of the organ participate but in which the liver cells themselves regenerate inadequately because the injurious stimulus persists. The result is functional liver failure, complications due to abnormal blood circulation through the organ and relative overgrowth of fibrous and biliary tissues.

One or two other examples of regeneration deserve mention. The inability of the skin epithelium, with certain exceptions, to reform specialised appendages has already been discussed. This incomplete adaptation does not apply to the mucous membrane of stomach and intestine, which after surgical removal will reconstitute all the original cell types, including highly specialised secretory epithelium. This is true also of the respiratory tract mucous membrane.

On the other side of the picture is the slow regeneration of the endothelium which line the large arteries such as the aorta. It may take months before a denuded area is fully lined by these cells, in sharp contrast to the exuberant proliferation of apparently identical capillary endothelium in regenerating connective tissue. Surgeons accelerate the reformation of the aortic lining after excision of diseased segments by inserting 'Dacron' ® grafts. The synthetic material provides a framework for organised blood clot which contains capillary endothelium and it may be these which supply a new source of aortic endothelium. The alveoli of the lung are lined by fairly simple cell types but regeneration after excision or damage is minimal except perhaps in young children. These discrepancies in regenerative powers provide good food for speculation but scientists have found it difficult to devise experiments that might explain them.

Healing of bones

Fractured bones heal in much the same way as subcutaneous tissue. The broken area fills with blood clot which is removed by mononuclear phagocytes (macrophages) (Fig. 11.15). Blood vessels grow into the area followed by migrating osteoblasts. These are a specialised form of fibroblast derived by proliferation of osteoblasts in the periosteum, the membrane covering the bone surface. The osteoblasts secrete collagen and muco-polysaccharides, known collectively in this context as osteoid (Fig. 11.16). Minerals are deposited in this material as apatite complexes of calcium, phosphate and magnesium. This mass of calcified tissue is known as the provisional callus. It is quickly remodelled by phagocytic giant cells called osteoclasts, which are

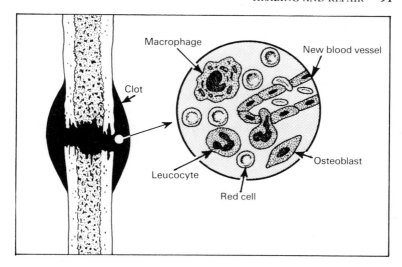

Fig. 11.15 Early events in healing of a fracture.

probably a form of multinucleate macrophage and at the same time the bone is reconstructed to recover its final form complete with Haversian canals and related structures.

Factors influencing wound healing

Generally speaking wound healing is an efficient process whose

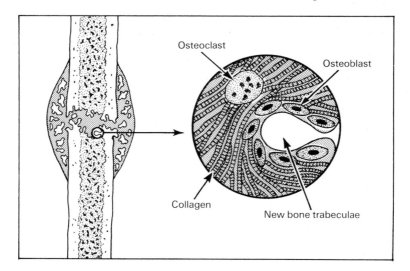

Fig. 11.16 Later events in healing of a fracture.

progress it is hard to arrest. There are factors, however, which can interfere with almost any stage. If the scavenging phase is disturbed healing will be slow. The commonest cause is persistent active inflammation due for example to bacterial infection. This provides new exudate faster than the macrophages can remove it, or may replace the macrophages with polymorphonuclear leucocytes, or may damage the macrophages by action of bacterial toxins, or interfere with their phagocytosis of debris by blocking the phagocytic receptor sites on their surface with immunoglobulin plus bacterial antigen.

The ingrowth of blood vessels and fibroblasts *per se* is probably seldom directly interfered with. It is commonly stated that corticosteroids used in therapy do so, but this is doubtful. If these drugs do delay wound healing it is more likely to be attributable to an effect on macrophage phagocytosis.

However, a reasonably good blood supply is essential for wound healing since the actively metabolising site needs oxygen and substrates to provide it with energy, and new blood vessels must reach it from a patent adjacent microcirculation. Excess movement of the damaged wound edges will obviously slow the remodelling process and in fractured bones is a particularly serious handicap to a good result.

Chemical factors may interfere with wound healing. Lack of ascorbic acid (vitamin C) prevents the hydroxylation of proline and thus makes it impossible to synthesise mature cross-linked collagen, although protocollagen accumulates. Toxic alkaloids causing the disease of lathyrism also prevent proper cross linking of collagen fibres and there are rare metabolic diseases of man and animals with similar effects. Simple malnutrition does not prevent wound healing but there is evidence that trace elements, notably zinc, may be required in high amounts for optimal healing and that occasionally dietary supplements may accelerate the process.

Bibliography

Gardner D L (ed) 1978 Diseases of connective tissue. Royal College of Pathologists, London

Kernahan D A, Vistnes L M (eds) 1977 Biological Aspects of Reconstructive Surgery. Little Brown, Boston

Maibach H I, Rovee D T (eds) 1972 Epidermal wound healing. Year Book Medical Publishers, New York

Ross R, Everett N B, Tyler R 1970 Wound healing and collagen formation VI. The origin of the wound fibroblast; studies in parabiosis. Journal of Cell Biology 44: 645

12

The systemic response to injury: reaction of the bone marrow

In pathology the word 'injury' embraces every form of tissue damage including bacterial or viral infection, chemical or thermal insult or mechanical destruction of body tissues by accident or by deliberate violence, the latter category including surgical operations. Even trivial injury produces a local reaction of the surviving tissues, i.e. inflammation (p. 58). More serious injury is accompanied also by a systemic reaction in which the cardiovascular system, the endocrine system and indeed the whole bodily metabolism are involved. The knowledge we possess of these responses has been accumulated mainly from research initiated in time of war when information was necessary to reduce battle casualties.

Injury as defined above is the main threat to those individuals young enough to hold the responsibility for reproducing the species. It is predictable therefore that the systemic reaction to injury as described in the pages which follow consists largely of compensatory mechanisms which must have been selected for by evolutionary pressures.

Red blood corpuscles

When blood is lost from the body (haemorrhage) in large amounts, either acutely, i.e. for a short period or chronically, i.e. in smaller amounts over a long period, the red cell precursors in the bone marrow react appropriately. Red cell production (erythropoesis) is regulated by a refined system involving a hormone, erythropoetin, partly produced in the kidney. When there is a need for more oxygen, e.g. at high altitudes, the marrow puts out more oxygen-binding haemoglobin by producing additional red blood corpuscles. After massive haemorrhage there is a transient drop in the number of circulating red cells but this deficiency is soon made good provided that adequate amounts of iron (part of the haemoglobin molecule) and other nutritional factors are available. In chronic blood loss, e.g. from a bleeding peptic ulcer or excessive menstrual bleeding, it is common for the dietary intake of iron to be inadequate and for an iron-deficiency type of anaemia (shortage of haemoglobin) to result. There are of course a number of diseases such as pernicious anaemia, affecting the red cell precursors in the bone marrow but these are the province of the haematologist and do not fall within the scope of general pathology. As regards the general reaction to injury the essential point is that a successful humoral feedback system regulates red cell production and returns it to normal levels, without over-reacting. The main constraints in the adaptive process which prevent over-reaction are the high daily output of red cells and the resultant very great demand on the essential ingredients in their manufacture, especially iron, which quickly becomes a limiting factor because any increase in its absorption from the diet is difficult to achieve and because the body's stores are small.

Platelets

Obviously the major effect of injury on the bone marrow is to create a demand for replacement of blood cells lost by haemorrhage to the exterior or into damaged tissues. In the case of red cells this need is met by positive feedback mediated by erythropoetin. A similar mechanism operates in the case of platelets. Numerous experiments have demonstrated the appearance in the plasma of platelet-depleted animals of a substance which induces increased platelet production. This presumably operates on the megakaryocyte, the bone marrow precursor of platelets. Unlike the comparable erythropoesis there is usually an overproduction of platelets by up to 50 per cent over normal circulating values and this has its dangers since it may lead to undesirable effects, i.e. thrombosis (p. 140). The substance which stimulates platelet formation after injury is called thrombopoetin and, although it withstands boiling, it appears to be a protein or peptide. Its source of manufacture and storage in the body is uncertain but the kidney and the spleen both seem to have been excluded. If the nature of the injury is such as to consume platelets faster than they can be replaced, a deficiency of platelets develops in the circulation (thrombocytopaenia). However this situation seldom occurs as a result merely of repeated haemorrhage so there is no direct parallel with red blood cells which become scarce under such circumstances due to shortage of iron. Platelet deficiency is usually due to disease of the bone marrow itself or to antibodies which destroy these cells in the blood as in Type II drug hypersensitivity. If as in some diseases, however, there is generalised coagulation of blood inside vessels with massive incorporation of platelets in the clot, persistent thrombocytopaenia may result. This will lead to further bleeding since platelets are needed for normal haemostasis and a progressive failure of adaptation typical of pathology will result.

Neutrophil polymorphs (granulocytes)

Any form of local tissue injury leading to exudation of polymorphs is likely to be associated with an increase in the number of these cells circulating in the blood (neutrophil leucocytosis, neutrophilia). The largest neutrophilia is seen usually during bacterial inflammation. Sterile inflammation as occurs in infarcted heart muscle (p. 153) has a similar but smaller effect on blood leucocytes. As an exception to the rule, one or two examples of bacterial inflammation, notably typhoid fever lead to a drop rather than a rise in numbers of circulating polymorphs. Virus-induced inflammation seldom causes a neutrophilia although there are exceptions such as poliomyelitis. In general there is a good correlation between the number of polymorphs exuding into the inflamed tissue site and the size of the accompanying leucocytosis. This suggests at once that leucocytosis is the result of a positive feedback mechanism and indeed there is convincing evidence in man and animals that both positive and negative feedback occurs. Positive feedback means that a deficiency of cells results in their increased production and negative feedback means that an excess of cells leads to a diminution in their production.

The kinetics of granulocytes are complicated because three compartments must be considered; the bone marrow, the blood and the tissues. In inflammation, in order to maintain a steady state there is a demand for mature neutrophils to replace those lost in the injured tissues (p. 60). This demand is met by maintaining the size of the total granulocyte pool. As we have seen, feedback mechanisms in pathology tend to over-react and the response to leucocyte loss is no exception. As a result of the exaggerated reaction the granulocyte pool usually increases to well beyond its normal size so that there is an excessive number of neutrophil polymorphonuclear leucocytes in the circulation, i.e. a neutrophil leucocytosis.

One result of this excess is that individual cells spend more time than usual in the blood stream (i.e. their half life or $T\frac{1}{2}$ is raised) because the augmented entry of leucocytes into the total blood granulocyte pool from the bone marrow is faster than their disappearance into the inflamed site. Nevertheless the absolute number of leucocytes replaced each day by fresh leucocytes from the marrow (the granulocyte turnover rate) is also raised.

The exaggerated increase in the size of the total blood granulocyte pool is of course achieved by an additional output of leucocytes from the bone marrow. The extra output is due largely to a release of mature leucocytes earlier than would normally occur. In addition the cell cycle time of the leucocyte precursors, i.e. the time needed to divide and produce mature leucocytes, is probably shortened. Under extreme conditions of leucocyte demand, immature forms escape into the blood but the more primitive leucocyte precursors only leave the bone marrow in primary disease of that organ such as leukaemia.

It is well known that various sorts of 'stress' such as physical exercise, fear, or even sitting for an examination induce a leucocytosis of neutrophils. This is due to release of extra amounts of adrenalin and of corticosteroid hormones from the adrenal cortex, the process being controlled from the pituitary gland and the hypothalamus of the brain. The kinetics of this situation differ from tissue injury in that although the total blood granulocyte pool is increased (Fig. 12.1), the granulocyte turnover rate remains normal because there is no increase in migration of leucocytes into the tissues. The granulocytosis of stress is due to release into the circulation of leucocytes sequestered along the walls of blood vessels throughout the body. This sequestration of 'marginated' granulocytes is normal and release of the cells leads to no change in the size of the bone marrow pool (Fig 12.1).

After injury a variety of endogenous substances appear in the circulation and cause a granulocytosis. Some of these act by inducing a premature release of mature polymorphs from the bone marrow. In this category comes the leucocytosis-inducing factor (LIF) which appears in the blood after injection of bacterial endotoxin or after destruction of leucocytes.

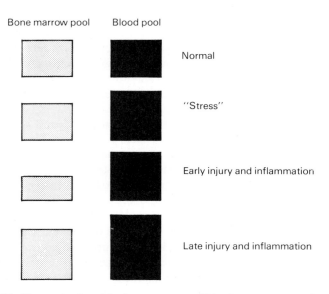

Fig. 12.1 Changes in size of the bone marrow and blood compartments of granulocytes after injury and 'stress'.

Table 12.1 Mechanisms of leucocytosis

Endogenous mediator	Mode of action
Adrenalin and other stress hormones	Release from tissue pool of marginated leucocytes
Leucocytosis-inducing factor (LIF) C3 fragment (leucocyte mobilising factor)	Release from pool of mature neutrophils in bone marrow
Colony-stimulating factor Inhibition of granulocyte chalone	Stimulation of mitosis in neutrophil precursors in bone marrow

Another substance which works in the same way and circulates after injury is a special fragment of the third component of complement (C3), known as the leucocyte-mobilising factor.

Another substance, colony-stimulating factor also appears in the circulation after injury or infection. This is a glycoprotein which stimulates mitosis in neutrophil precursors in the bone marrow and increases the size of the marrow pool. A similar effect could be produced by a granulocyte chalone (p. 88) if it were certain that one existed. These effects are set out in Table 12.1.

Monocytes

Although monocytes migrate freely into inflamed tissues especially if the process is prolonged (chronic inflammation) an excess of monocytes in the circulation is unusual. Nevertheless, a positive feedback mechanism has been demonstrated in which loss of these cells into peritoneal exudates is balanced by augmented production and release from the bone marrow. In mice the normal steady state monocyte production is about 0.6×10^5 cells per hour. In acute peritoneal inflammation the figure increases briefly to 1.0×10^5 cells per hour and the cell cycle time, i.e. the time needed for a monocyte precursor to divide and produce its progeny falls from 16 to 10 hours. The production rate of the monocyte precursor cell, the promonocyte, also shows a transient rise. The rate increases mainly because the DNA synthesis time, i.e. the 'S' phase of the mitotic cycle is shortened in the bone marrow cells. There is much less effect on the later parts of the mitotic cycle, i.e. 'GI', 'G2' and 'M'. Corticosteroids prevent these effects of inflammation on the bone marrow monocytes and to some extent therefore act in a contrary fashion to their effects on polymorphonuclear leucocytes (p. 96) although the details of this difference are not yet clear. The positive feedback for monocyte regulation may operate through a factor which appears in the circulation in acute inflammation and which when injected into normal mice causes a threefold rise in blood monocytes with no effect on granulocytes or lymphocytes.

Lymphocytes

Changes in numbers of circulating lymphocytes are not of major importance in the reaction to injury. The numbers may rise in a variety of virus infections and fall when output of adrenocortical hormones is elevated. In one virus disease (infectious mononucleosis) abnormal lymphocytes appear in the blood stream and their recognition by the pathologist helps to establish the diagnosis. Lymphocyte kinetics are of course very complex since there are at least two major sub-populations and a number of compartments in which they exist for widely differing lengths of time.

Eosinophils

This cell is a cousin of the neutrophil polymorphonuclear leucocyte with a similar life pattern. It originates in a bone marrow precursor cell, circulates in small numbers in the blood and enters the tissues freely. Its life span may be longer than that of the neutrophil polymorph. The eosinophil gets its name from the affinity of its lysosomal granules for eosin dyes but the significance of this staining is not known. The eosinophil appears in large numbers in two situations; infestation with worms and Type I hypersensitivity (p. 43). There is a link here with mast cells and with IgE (p. 28). Eosinophils probably cooperate with mast cells in the elimination from host tissues of certain worms (p. 44) and their mobilisation is probably assisted by sensitised lymphocytes exerting cell mediated immunity (p. 35). Eosinophilia may also occur as a by-product of the mast cell degranulation which occurs in both worm infestation and in Type I hypersensitivity although the mechanism of the link is not yet clear. Indeed, the properties of the eosinophils and the nature of their participation in these events also remains obscure. In general the increase in circulating eosinophils parallels their appearance in large numbers in sites of inflammation. No factor causing release of eosinophils from the marrow has been convincingly identified but it does seem that there are chemotactic substances which are partially specific for eosinophils at suitable sites of inflammation.

Bibliography

Golde D W, Cline M J 1974 regulation of granulopoesis. New England Journal of Medicine 291: 1388

Van Furth R (ed) 1975 Mononuclear phagocytes in immunity, infection and pathology. Blackwell, Oxford

Wickramasinghe S N 1975 Human bone marrow. Blackwell, Oxford

13

Fever

Fever is the elevation of body temperature above normal. Of all the general systemic accompaniments of injury it is the most widely and easily observed. The normal body temperature is about 37° C (98.4° F) and is usually measured by a thermometer inserted in mouth, rectum or axilla. Precise regulation of body temperature is a vital element in physiological homeostasis and is controlled for the most part through the skin. When it is necessary to lose heat, e.g. because heat has been produced through exercise, the skin vessels dilate and blood flow and heat loss increases via radiation. If this is insufficient the sweat glands are stimulated to lose heat by means of evaporation. Conversely, to gain heat, e.g. because of low environmental temperature, the skin vessels constrict and cutaneous blood flow and therefore heat loss via radiation is reduced. If it is necessary to generate heat there is repetitive contraction of muscle fibres causing shivering. All these physiological phenonema are reproduced during fever often in rapid succession, shivering under these circumstances being known as rigors. In pathology, however, the fever is due to an alteration of the setting of the centre in the brain, the thermoregulatory centre, which controls body temperature. Thus fever results from interference with the thermostat itself wheareas non-pathological temperature regulation is dependent upon environmental temperature and the amount of heat generated by the body's metabolism.

Fever can be deliberately induced in humans by injection of pyrogens, i.e. substances of biological origin, e.g. bacterial extracts, which cause fever. When this is done it is easy to show how contraction of skin vessels and reduction in blood flow in skin (causing a feeling of coldness) and shivering precede a rise in body temperature. Often the increase is overdone and there is a response of sweating, vasodilatation (with a feeling of being hot) followed in turn by a compensatory increase in heat loss. The changes in blood flow are dependent on the vasomotor nerves and fever is prevented if these nerves no longer function, e.g. in patients with damage high up in the spinal cord. In such cases the accompaniments of fever, notably headache, are also abolished. Thus it seems likely that headache is the result of the fever. Patients with non-functioning thermoregulatory centres do not become feverish if pyrogen is injected. Fever is therefore due to an action of fever-inducing substances on this brain centre and is brought about by the vasomotor nerves.

Animal experiments indicate that the site of the thermoregulatory centre is in the anterior hypothalamus and that it contains warm and cold receptors which are triggered off as appropriate. During fever they work with normal sensitivity but the threshold or set point at which they work is raised so that body heat is maintained at an abnormally high level.

The commonest injury causing fever is of course bacterial or viral infection and for some time now it has been possible to obtain purified chemical pyrogens from dead bacteria. When obtained from Gram-negative organisms such as *E. coli* or *Salm. abortus* (p. 6) these are known as endotoxin and consist of lipopolysaccharides. Many other bacterial species including Gram-positive cocci (p. 6) also yield pyrogens. However it is now thought unlikely that these are the direct cause of fever. Instead they act indirectly by causing the liberation from leucocytes of a quite different substance, a peptide of molecular weight between 10000—20000 daltons. This peptide is present in monocytes and polymorphonuclear leucocytes and is known therefore as endogenous or leucocytic pyrogen.

That bacterial pyrogen acts via endogenous pyrogen has been shown in various ways. The fever caused by injection of endotoxin takes some time, usually about 90 minutes, to develop (latent period) and after repeated injections does not develop at all (refractory period). Injection of endogenous pyrogen, however, leads to a much more rapid onset of fever usually within 15 minutes and repeated injections continue to take effect. If endogenous pyrogen is injected directly into the arteries supplying the hypothalamic thermoregulatory centre fever develops more quickly than when the pyrogen is given via the peripheral veins, e.g. in a limb. Bacterial pyrogen, however, exerts its effect no more quickly when administered into the hypothalamic vessels than into these veins. The two types of pyrogen can be distinguished by tests such as heating. Endogenous pyrogen is very easily destroyed by heating whereas bacterial pyrogen remains active after being incubated at 170°C. Study of the blood of animals and man suffering from bacterial or viral induced fever shows that it is endogenous pyrogen which is circulating and that the amount varies directly with the height of the temperature. Finally, adding bacterial pyrogen to normal leucocytes outside the body induces the cells to form and release endogenous pyrogen.

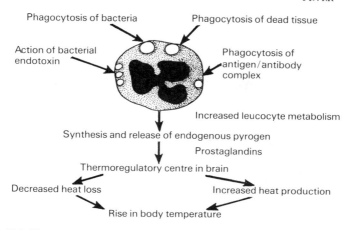

Fig. 13.1 The central role of the granulocyte in the mechanism of fever.

Normal leucocytes collected from blood do not contain endogenous pyrogen whereas leucocytes harvested from inflammatory exudates do so, indicating that injury makes the cells synthesise the substance. As we have seen this injury-associated stimulus can be bacterial endotoxin but in fact phagocytosis of any type of particle will switch on the mechanism (Fig. 13.1). The mechanism itself consists of two parts, synthesis of the endogenous pyrogen, easily suppressed by inhibitors of respiration or protein synthesis and its release, which is prevented with much more difficulty. Clearly the burst of metabolic activity which occurs in leucocytes after phagocytosis (p. 23) is partly concerned with pyrogen synthesis.

Although the terms leucocytic and endogenous pyrogen tend to be used as synonyms, there are other bodily substances which produce fever on injection. Certain corticosteroids have this property, notably aetiocholanolone which is a steroid degradation product. Aetiocholanolone probably exerts its effect by causing release of leucocytic pyrogen. Noradrenalin causes fever at least in some mammalian species, especially when injected directly into the hypothalamus. Finally, the prostaglandins, notably PGE[1] (p. 65) will induce fever on injection. Their mode of action is not yet clear and they could work by inducing leucocytes to release pyrogen, or by stimulating noradrenalin release in the hypothalamus or directly on the hypothalamic receptors themselves. At the moment the evidence favours the view that prostaglandins act directly on the hypothalamus and that endogenous pyrogen may cause fever by inducing synthesis and release of prostaglandins in the brain. This would of course explain the antipyretic action of drugs such as aspirin which are powerful inhibitors of prostaglandin synthesis and release. The ultimate mode of action of pyrogens on nerve cells is obviously not yet clear but it is likely that local ionic movements are involved, a rise in sodium leading to fever and a rise in calcium to its disappearance. The cause of the sensation of ill-being (malaise) which usually accompanies fever is uncertain. It may be a direct consequence of pyrexia or could possibly result from an independent action of prostaglandins on some part of the brain.

A usual companion of fever is an increase in the heart rate, so that taking the pulse is usually combined with taking the temperature in the solemn bedside ritual of the doctor's visit. The increased heart rate (tachycardia) indicates an increased cardiac output which is very closely linked to a rise in body temperature. It is not certain how these two events are related, but it is known that if fever is prevented by damage to the nervous pathways in the spinal cord, cardiac output too, fails to rise. On the other hand, the two phenomena may be disassociated as in typhoid fever when the temperature is raised but the pulse is slow.

There is little information on the benefit, if any, of fever to the patient. It would be justifiable to suspect that because the reaction is so widespread in mammalian species, it must have been selected for. It is often suggested that the mechanisms of defence against infection function better at a temperature above normal but here again there is lack of supporting data. The one useful function of which we can be certain is that fever enables an observer to detect the presence of infection in another individual and thus to isolate him. For the many mammals which live in packs or colonies this could have survival value for the species if not for the individual. For the individual mammal self-recognition of fever, followed by early self-regulated rest would in some cases at least determine a favourable outcome to an infection.

Bibliography

Atkins E, Bodel G 1974 Fever, In: Zweifach B W, Grant L, McCluskey R T (ed) The inflammatory response, p 467. Academic Press, New York
Lomax P, Schönbaum E (eds) 1979 Body Temperature; regulation, drug effects and therapeutic implications. Marcel Dekker, New York

14

Changes in plasma proteins after injury

After injury, and its associated local inflammatory reaction, character-istic changes occur in some of the plasma proteins. These changes are evident as increased blood concentration of the proteins concerned but actually represent alterations in liver cell metabolism, since apart from immunoglobulins, plasma proteins are manufactured in that organ.

One of the most consistent features is an elevation in the level of circulating fibrinogen and increased synthesis of this protein by the liver. This probably represents an exaggerated positive feedback response to loss of fibrinogen in the exudate from inflamed blood vessels (p. 61) or in the course of haemorrhage.

Fibrinogen is a high molecular weight protein and when large molecules appear in the plasma in excessive amounts the red corpus-cles clump together to form heavy rouleaux. This is seldom evident inside the body but if a sample of such blood is removed, prevented from clotting and allowed to sediment under gravity, the red cells will settle much faster than normal. This erythrocyte sedimentation rate is easily measured and forms a useful and simple bedside index of the presence and severity of inflammation, although it will be raised by an excess of any high molecular weight substance in the plasma, so that in a few rare instances it will be due to a primary abnormality of the plasma proteins.

Besides fibrinogen, other plasma proteins made in the liver also appear in excess in the blood after injury and some of them may not be demonstrable at all in normal people. These are the acute phase proteins, mostly α_2 globulins. The best known of these is C-reactive protein, so called because it reacts with the carbohydrate of pneumococci. This substance can activate the complement pathway but its appearance is something of a mystery. It has recently been found in the serum of normal fish, plaice to be more precise, in which it may act as an opsonin, aiding phagocytosis of micro-organisms (p. 19) pathogenic for aquatic creatures. Its presence in man might therefore be a phylogenetic hangover. Other acute phase proteins possess modest anti-inflammatory properties and may help to termi-

103

nate and thereby control inflammatory reactions. In its reaction to injury the liver also synthesises more lipoprotein and more microsomal detoxifying enzymes (p. 158).

It seems therefore that injury stimulates the liver not only to replace protein lost into sites of damage but also to a selective excess production of certain other proteins. These proteins appear in general to have survival value for the host but benefit may in some cases be demonstrable only in more primitive vertebrates such as fish, in which antibodies are slow to appear after infection.

Blood coagulation after injury

Reference has already been made to the elevation in blood fibrinogen levels and in platelet numbers (p. 94) which occur within two to four days and one to three weeks after injury respectively. These changes, reflected in a raised erythrocyte sedimentation rate and a propensity to venous thrombosis (p. 143) are accompanied by complex and poorly understood alterations in the coagulability of the blood. Initially, there is usually an increased tendency for clotting which is certainly desirable for the patient since blood vessels may have been severed. After a few hours, however, blood coagulation becomes slowed and the dissolution of clotted fibrin by the blood enzyme fibrinolysin is also retarded. The partial failure of blood clotting is reflected in the old observation that in patients dying after severe injury the blood remains fluid after death instead of clotting as is usual.

The diminished powers of blood clotting seen after injury are associated with falls in all the factors concerned in the process. Platelet numbers drop and there is a measurable decline in the concentrations of prothrombin, plasminogen and clotting factors such as V, VII and X. The key to these changes probably lies in the paradoxical observation that in animals, administration of the anti-clotting substance heparin prevents them. This suggests that the fall in clotting factors is due to their consumption in intravascular coagulation and that if the latter is prevented, hypocoagulability after injury will not develop. Evidence that this is the case comes from the observations that fibrinogen levels may also fall and that fibrin degradation products appear in blood and urine. In addition, microthrombi are frequently found in the lungs of such patients and less commonly major thrombi in arteries and veins (p. 140). This complication is known as disseminated intravascular coagulation (DIC). The unpleasant combination of inappropriate blood clotting, platelet aggregation and fibrin breakdown and eventual failure of blood coagulation is described elsewhere (p. 105) and is due to activation of the complicated system of interlocking mediators described in Chapter 10.

Bibliography for Chapter 14 appears on p. 115.

15

Other changes in the plasma proteins

Fibrinogen

This is the precursor of fibrin, the final product of the almost absurdly elaborate blood coagulation cascade. Its role and the rise in its concentration following injury and inflammation are discussed elsewhere (p. 103). A fall in blood fibrinogen levels is a serious matter because it may lead to fatal haemorrhage. The most important pathological situation in which this occurs is known as diffuse intravascular coagulation (DIC) or consumptive coagulopathy. DIC is caused by the release of clotting factors into the circulation. This occurs in amniotic fluid embolism during parturition, or after severe injury or widespread damage to endothelium (p. 104), e.g. by bacterial endotoxin. The result is the formation of innumerable fibrin thrombi in tiny blood vessels. Because of this fibrinogen is consumed faster than the liver can re-synthesise it. To make matters worse, the massive fibrin formation activates the fibrinolysin enzyme system involving conversion of blood plasminogen to plasmin. By enzyme action the fibrin is partially digested with the formation of fibrin degradation products (FDP) which are peptides. FDP have the property of inhibiting fibrin formation which is not surprising, since it is a general rule in chemistry that the products of a reaction tend to inhibit that reaction. The results for the patient, however, are unfortunate, because he or she now not only lacks the substrate to permit clotting but has in addition an excess of inhibitors of the clotting process itself. The consequence is massive and often fatal haemorrhage of which the classical example is the uncontrollable postpartum haemorrhage previously seen in obstetrics. Happily, transfusion of fibrinogen and fresh blood normally brings this vicious cycle to an end.

On other occasions, a similar situation arises without intravascular coagulation, due mainly to massive activation of the fibrinolytic system, i.e. of the enzyme plasmin. This may occur after severe injury and is due to release into the circulation of an activator of plasmin present in tissues. Plasmin digests fibrinogen as well as fibrin so once again there is lack of fibrinogen coupled with excess of anticoagulant fibrin degradation products and massive haemorrhage is the result.

The globulins

These are usually subdivided by their electrophoretic mobility, i.e. alpha, beta or gamma. The globulins include the lipoproteins, discussed elsewhere (p. 133). Their other major role in pathology is their capacity as antibodies or immunoglobulins (p. 27). Changes in their blood concentration are tightly linked with the pathology of the lymphoid system which synthesises them. Hypogammaglobulinaemia may occur as a genetic disease in the first 6 months of life or develop later. As might be expected it leads to a greatly increased susceptibility to bacterial infection. A rise in immunoglobulin level is most usually seen in malignant disease of the lymphoid system, especially a form affecting the bone marrow, i.e. myelomatosis. A single cell line or clone of plasma cells (myeloma cells) undergoes malignant transformation and produces as might be predicted from the clonal selection theory of antibody formation (p. 38) a monoclonal antibody (M protein) which may reach very high levels in the plasma. The protein contains one heavy chain and one light chain (p. 29) and the light chains are often excreted in the urine (Bence-Jones protein). Myelomatosis is not common but is of great interest to immunologists and our knowledge of the immunoglobulin molecule has been greatly aided by this experiment of nature. The importance of the disease to scientists is likely to grow, because it is now possible to persuade myeloma cells in cell culture to produce a single, pure, monoclonal antibody to an antigen of one's choice. This is achieved by hybridising human myeloma cells with spleen cells from mice previously immunised by the investigator with his chosen antigen.

Amyloid

Amyloid is a substance which in the disease of amyloidosis, is deposited often in large amounts in and around the small blood vessels and sinusoids of liver, spleen, kidney, gastrointestinal tract and lymph nodes or within the myocardium, or respiratory tract. It acquired its name because its staining properties wrongly suggested that it was of a starchy nature. The electron microscope reveals amyloid to consist of innumerable, interlacing fine fibrils giving a highly characteristic appearance. Chemical analysis of these insoluble fibrils has proved difficult but there is no doubt that amyloid is a protein. Amino-acid sequencing indicates that amyloid is derived partly from fragments of the variable portion of the light chain of immunoglobulins and partly from fragments of an abnormal circulating protein (SAA) found only in amyloidosis. Immunoglobulins are not fibrillar proteins but suitable partial digestion of their light chains has produced fragments which undergo spontaneous transformation into fibrils. This fibrillogenic potential is probably possessed by a number of immunoglobulin degradation products and presumably also by those derived from the circulating protein (SAA) peculiar to amyloid. The peculiar amyloid protein has a stereotyped and unusual amino acid composition whereas that of the immunoglobulin component of amyloid is much more variable.

The commonest cause of amyloidosis used to be long-standing infections such as tuberculosis or syphilis and it is still seen now in such circumstances. More usually nowadays it is seen as a complication of diseases associated with abnormalities of the immunological or lymphoid system, e.g. rheumatoid arthritis, Hodgkins disease or myelomatosis. In addition, the disease appears in horses used for repeated production of antibody for the preparation of antitoxins.

It seems likely that amyloid deposition is a consequence of abnormal production of at least two proteins. One of these (SAA) seems to belong to the general category of 'acute phase proteins' (p. 103). produced by the liver after injury. The other is abnormal immunoglobulin. Both give rise to degradation products and in most cases of amyloid, both 'primary' and 'secondary' (to other diseases), both proteins are present in the deposits. Why fibril-forming degradation products should accumulate is not clear. Nor is it known whether they simply leak through vessel walls and then precipitate in the wall or just outside it or whether the fibril-provoking degradation occurs within mononuclear phagocytes which then discharge their contents or disintegrate around them. It is strange that although the fibrils of amyloid are remarkably uniform in their ultrastructural appearance, they are usually composed of at least two quite different proteins.

Albumin

This is the largest single component of the plasma proteins. It is unusual for its concentration to rise significantly, but a number of diseases lead to a fall in its concentration (hypoalbuminaemia). This is important because it is the major source of oncotic pressure in the circulation and a fall leads to serious imbalance in the forces controlling fluid shift between vessels and tissues. Thus a serious decline in plasma albumin concentration is likely to lead to a diminished plasma volume and to the implementation of homeostatic mechanisms, such as water and sodium retention which, in pathological as opposed to normal physiological circumstances, lead to oedema (p. 174).

A severe drop in plasma albumin levels occurs commonly in

advanced liver disease, such as cirrhosis. Indeed albumin synthesis seems a rather sensitive indicator of liver cell damage. Albumin is involved in the transport of fatty acids and the appearance of lipid accumulation in the early stages of impaired hepatic function may be partly attributable to defective albumin synthesis.

The other major cause of a striking fall in circulating albumin is massive loss of the protein in the urine. This is seen most clearly in a form of renal dysfunction known as the nephrotic syndrome. This occurs in a variety of glomerular diseases in which the main effect is to render the glomerulus highly permeable to plasma protein. Permeability often varies inversely with molecular weight, so that albumin, being the smallest of the plasma proteins, is most readily lost in the urine.

Starvation leads to lowered concentrations of plasma albumin and it is a fine point whether this is due to direct lack of the constituent amino acids or to impaired liver function of nutritional origin. In either case, in spite of the prevalence of alcoholic liver disease in the West, on a world-wide basis malnutrition must be by far the commonest cause of hypoalbuminaemia.

Hyperlipoproteinaemia

Lipid is present in the blood plasma as free fatty acids, cholesterol, cholesterol esters, triglycerides and sundry phospholipids and caretenoids. All are bound to some protein moiety and as a group constitute the lipoproteins. Free fatty acids are transported mainly in combination with plasma albumin, but the remainder are bound chiefly to various globulins. Thus alpha-lipoprotein incorporates phospholipid and free fatty acids. Beta-lipoprotein contains cholesterol. Pre-beta lipoprotein carries triglyceride in fasting individuals. Chylomicrons include all three globulins and carry triglyceride obtained from the diet. The terms alpha, beta and pre-beta refer to the relative positions of the lipoproteins on electrophoresis. Of importance in pathology is the relative flotation density of the proteins which depends on the quantity and type of lipid they incorporate. Alpha-protein is a high density lipoprotein (HDL), beta-lipoprotein is low density lipoprotein (LDL) and pre-beta lipoprotein is very low density lipoprotein (VLDL).

It is now realised that it is quite common for individuals to have blood concentrations of one or more of the lipoproteins which exceed normal values. These abnormalities have been classified into six main sub-groups. The importance of the classification is that hyperlipidaemia is one of the main causes of the early onset of atheroma but that not all types of hyperlipoproteinaemia have this lethal association.

Type I hyperlipidaemia is associated with raised amounts of

circulating chylomicrons and hence of triglyceride. It is familial but the high blood lipid levels depend upon a high intake of dietary fat. It does not appear to predispose to atheroma.

Type IIa hyperlipidaemia is a form of familial metabolic disease in which there are very high levels of circulating beta-lipoprotein and therefore of cholesterol. It is also known as familial hypercholestro-laemia. It has a strong association with early-onset atheroma and with a high mortality from ischaemic heart disease.

Type IIb hyperlipidaemia exhibits raised levels of both pre-Beta and beta-lipoprotein in the circulation. This sub-group is related to a high dietary intake of saturated animal fats and cholesterol. It also predisposes to early atheromatous disease.

Type III hyperlipidaemia indicates the presence of an abnormal lipoprotein containing both triglyceride and cholesterol. It locates in the beta range ('broad beta') and has a lower density than beta-lipoprotein. Nevertheless this group has not yet been shown to be at special risk from atheroma.

Type IV hyperlipidaemia exhibits raised levels of circulating pre-beta-lipoprotein and hence of triglyceride. It is linked with high dietary intake of carbohydrate and in the presence of such a diet strongly predisposes to an early onset of atheroma.

Type V hyperlipidaemia is the sub-group in which there is an excess of both chylomicrons and pre-beta lipoproteins in the circulation. It does not appear to be especially dangerous in precipitating early atheroma.

It is of interest that although all the above six categories are examples of familial hyperlipidaemia, two of them at least, i.e. types IIb and IV depend on a high dietary intake of fat or carbohydrate. They could be regarded as a genetically determined exaggerated response to a normal Western diet. This also means, however, that the hyperlipidaemia and hence the risk of early onset atheromatous disease can be diminished by dietary control.

In addition to the primary hyperlipidaemias discussed above, the phenomenon occurs as secondary hyperlipidaemia in other diseases. The most notable of them is diabetes mellitus (p. 226) in which levels of pre-beta-lipoproteins and chylomicrons tend to be elevated.

Bibliography

Frederickson D et al 1978 The familial hyperlipidaemias: in Stanbury J B et al (eds) The Metabolic Basis of Inherited Disease, McGraw-Hill, New York

Pras M, Gafin J 1977 The nature of amyloid. In Glynn L E, Steward M W (eds) Immunochemistry an advanced textbook. Wiley, New York p 509

The classification of hyperlipidaemias and hyperproteinaemies, 1970. W.H.O. Bulletin 43: 891

16

Endocrine and metabolic response to injury

Injury of all sorts but especially massive trauma, burns, haemorrhage or severe infection lead to activation of the hypothalamic – pituitary – adrenal axis. The first step is the arrival at the hypothalamic region of the brain of a variety of nervous and chemical stimuli from the area of damage. This causes the liberation from the hypothalamus of releasing factors which stimulate the anterior pituitary gland to free various hormones, notably ACTH (adrenocorticotropic hormone), but also growth hormone, thyroid stimulating hormone and probably others. A major result of anterior pituitary activation is stimulation of the adrenal cortex to release corticosteroid hormones. The role of these hormones in the general reaction to injury appears to be permissive rather than active. In other words, in the absence of adrenal cortex the animal dies after injury but quite small amounts of circulating hormone are sufficient to allow the usual reactions to develop and for the animal to survive. It is thought therefore that corticoids are necessary mainly to permit various other hormones and enzymes to work.

Apart from the basic need for adrenocortical hormones, the most important part of the endocrine reaction to general injury appears to be played by the adrenal medulla. This is of course part of the sympathetic nervous system, well known since the pioneer work of Cannon, to be activated by all sorts of stress and injury. The medulla itself secretes adrenalin and noradrenalin and these probably play an important role in the metabolic and vascular changes that occur after injury (p. 113) as well as in phenomena such as a minor leucocytosis (p. 95). The stimulus for this secretion is now thought to come from the receptors which monitor a fall in blood volume. This arrangement is appropriate since diminished blood volume (hypovolaemia) is the major common denominator in severe injury.

Metabolic response to injury
Striking metabolic changes are seen after many types of injury and can be followed in patients recovering from major surgical operations. The

changes affect carbohydrates, lipid and protein metabolism, and fall into three categories each seen at one characteristic stage after injury. There is the initial or ebb phase in which, mainly in response to adrenalin and noradrenalin secretion, there is increased breakdown of muscle glycogen to lactate and thence to glucose. There is also breakdown of fat deposits. These changes, due to activation of cyclic AMP, phosphorylase and lipase, are manifest in the blood as increased levels of glucose and fatty acids. By these means injury is quickly followed by mobilisation of readily utilised energy sources.

If injury is very severe and treatment unsuccessful the patient may enter the shock or necrobiotic phase of metabolic change (Fig. 16.1). As a result of inadequate perfusion of the tissues due to circulatory failure there is diminished oxygen consumption and sometimes a resultant fall in body temperature. Glucose utilisation is increased under these anaerobic conditions and there is a resultant fall in blood glucose concentration with an accumulation of lactate, leading to acidosis and death. Underperfusion of individual organs concerned with metabolic and hormonal regulation may lead to massive metabolic disturbance, the liver being the most notable example.

Most cases never enter the necrobiotic stage but some days after injury pass from the initial stage to the period of recovery or flow phase. During this period there is increased oxygen consumption and a rise in body temperature due to increased heat production. This is in turn due to increased oxidation of protein and protein catabolism manifest by increased urinary excretion of urea, sulphur, phosphorus

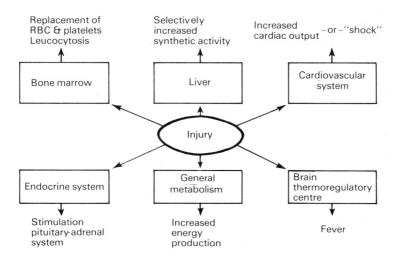

Fig. 16.1 The effects of tissue injury on various body systems.

and potassium. There is also increased turnover of glucose, and hyperglycaemia may develop. The picture is essentially one of enhanced glucose utilisation and gluconeogenesis using the labile protein stored in skeletal muscle as an energy source. Presumably the energy so generated is of use in restoring bodily function to normal. Protein catabolism is particularly dramatic and is partly due to a failure of the homeostatic mechanisms which normally preserve muscle protein at the expense of fat. One such failure is the inappropriate secretion of insulin which helps to block lipolysis. The enormous calorie requirement of severely injured patients losing bodily fuel in such large amounts has only recently been realised. Its balanced replacement often leads to remarkable recovery.

Electrolyte metabolism
Injury may be associated with particular loss of water and electrolytes, e.g. by vomiting, diarrhoea, haemorrhage or massive exudation of fluid into injured tissues. Quite apart from these possibilities, however, injury *per se* is accompanied by electrolyte changes, especially in sodium ions. The usual observation is of reduced sodium and enhanced potassium excretion in the urine, i.e. sodium retention. This is accompanied by a paradoxical fall in plasma sodium concentration. Sodium retention may sometimes be due to secretion of antidiuretic hormone (ADH) from the pituitary or to aldosterone secretion from the adrenal cortex both in response to hypovolaemia. There may also be enhanced reabsorption of sodium in the ascending limb of the loop of Henle due to diminished circulatory perfusion of the kidney, again consequent upon hypovolaemia. The paradoxical fall in serum sodium concentration is usually attributed to its entry into tissue cells as a result of disturbance of cellular metabolism.

17

The response of the circulation to injury

Generalised collapse of the patient after severe injury is commonly known as 'shock' and although the term is often loosely used it should really refer to the state of circulatory failure that is seen in these circumstances. The failure is due to a reduction in blood volume (hypovolaemia) relative to the capacity of the peripheral circulation. It results from haemorrhage or from loss of blood or plasma into damaged tissues or tissue spaces. Thus burned skin, crushed muscle or an infected peritoneal cavity are all effective in attracting a massive leakage of fluid from the circulation. As a result of hypovolaemia there is a fall in venous return to the heart and a fall in right atrial pressure leading to diminished cardiac output. Circulatory failure may be aggravated by increased blood viscosity due to loss of fluid. In most cases transfusion with blood plasma or plasma substitutes is effective but sometimes the patient fails to respond (irreversible shock). This is most commonly due to inadequate replacement of blood or plasma but sometimes probably results from persistent myocardial failure in which poor coronary blood flow may be a major factor. The small haemorrhages and areas of necrosis that are sometimes seen in the heart muscle of injured patients may be the result of this diminished blood supply.

A factor which is of major importance is lung function. The lungs may be underperfused by blood due to the fall in cardiac output and under-ventilated due perhaps to congestion, oedema (p. 174) and collapse of alveoli. These pulmonary changes may be due not only to diminished cardiac output but also to fat embolism with liberation of irritant fatty acids (p. 114), or to release of vasoactive peptides (kinins, p. 64). The major common pathway in this situation, known as 'shock lung' is probably oedema of the pulmonary interstitial tissue, especially the alveolar walls

Shock in overwhelming bacterial infections requires special mention. Sometimes there is obvious hypovolaemia as in the intense diarrhoea of cholera or in peritonitis. Sometimes, however, there is no apparent fluid loss, e.g. in septicaemia with Gram negative enterobacilli (endotoxin shock). There is usually diminished cardiac output, perhaps due to a direct effect on the myocardium of bacterial toxins. The lungs may also suffer and show major disturbances in both perfusion and ventilation, the mechanism again being uncertain. Clearly, in all forms of shock once the tissues begin to suffer from a lack of oxygen there will tend to be a progressive failure of adaptation. This is especially true of the organs responsible for a supply of oxygenated blood, namely the heart and lungs. Whatever happens later, in the heart and brain, poor circulatory response to sympathomimetic stimulation at first preserves blood supply.

In most tissues, oxygen lack is aggravated by particular reductions in arterial blood supply. The most notable example is the kidney where vasoconstriction may combine with reduced cardiac output to cause renal ischaemia (lack of blood supply) severe enough to result in death and disintegration of tubules. The vasoconstriction, also seen in skeletal muscle and in the liver and intestines, is sometimes described teleologically as an attempt to divert blood to the immediately essential organs of heart, lungs and brain. If so, it is demonstrably unsuccessful and better thought of as part of the complex haemodynamic pattern of shock. It may produce its own ill effects such as renal failure and also bowel-wall ischaemia leading to the massive escape into the circulation of intestinal organisms. It therefore illustrates the dictum that disease is the resultant of the direct effects of injury, in this case hypovolaemia, and of the reaction to injury, e.g. renal ischaemia.

There is a large literature devoted to experimental models of shock especially to the causes of irreversibility such as damage to the intestinal wall or failure of the mononuclear phagocyte system. There is general agreement, however, that these laboratory simulations have only dubious relevance to the human condition.

Fat embolism

Severe trauma, especially involving fractures of the long bones, is quite commonly associated with fat embolism in which globules of neutral fat lodge in the lungs and sometimes in the brain and skin. An embolus is any circulating particle whose passage through the arteries is arrested by its size. In fat embolism there is impaired functioning of the brain and the lungs and death may ensue. Until recently it was generally accepted that the source of the fat emboli was the marrow fat of the injured bones. There is now a powerful school of thought which holds that the emboli are aggregations of the fatty particles called chylomicrons which are already in the blood as a natural constituent, perhaps induced to coalesce by concomitant intravascular clumping of platelets. The evidence is not conclusive either way and both theories may be true.

The most pronounced feature of fat embolism is a lowered oxygen concentration in the arterial blood. This is associated with striking changes in the lungs, ranging from congestion to oedema, collapse and haemorrhage. Presumably these changes interfere with oxygenation of the blood and the discharge of carbon dioxide. It is not yet clear to what extent they are due to mechanical blockage of the vessels by fat or to liberation in the lung of irritants such as free fatty acids, prostaglandins or kinins. A similar obscurity surrounds the mechanism of the brain anoxia which is seen. Some of this may be attributable to mechanical blockage of brain blood vessels by fat emboli which have passed through the lung. Some symptoms and signs of cerebral dysfunction may, however, merely reflect lack of oxygen in the blood, since of all body cells those of the central nervous system are most susceptible to anoxia.

Bibliography *(Chapters 14, 16 17)*

Haberland G L, Lewis D H (eds) 1973 The lung in shock. Schattouer Verlag, Stuttgart

Harper H A 1977 In: Kernahan D A, Vistnes L M (eds) Biological aspects of reconstrutive surgery Little Brown, Boston, p 75

Hunt A (ed) 1972 Pathology of injury. Harvey Miller & Medcalf, Aylesbury

Wilkinson A W, Cuthbertson D 1977 Metabolism and the response to injury. Pitman, Tunbridge Wells

18

Chronic inflammation

When an inflammatory response lasts long enough to extend over a year or more it is termed chronic. Sometimes the process is merely a succession of attacks of acute inflammation, and in these cases the patient suffers recurrent bouts of pain and fever, and microscopical examination of the affected tissues shows changes not very different from those of non-recurrent acute inflammation, although there may be evidence of healing between attacks. Organs prone to this type of chronic inflammation are the gall bladder, kidney and large intestine.

The other type of chronic inflammation has a less obvious connection with acute inflammation in that the cardinal signs of redness, heat and pain are often absent and in that the microscopical picture also is different, with dense masses of cells instead of oedema, fibrin and polymorphs. The compact nature of these lesions led to the idea that they were some sort of tumour and to their being named granulomas, that is to say tumours of granular appearance. The discovery that some granulomas were caused by bacteria, e.g. tuberculosis, leprosy and syphilis and later the discovery of the nature of the constituent cells of the granuloma revealed their inflammatory nature. Like other examples of inflammation, granulomas originate in a local reaction to injury of the microcirculation and its contents. The special character of granulomatous inflammation lies largely in the important role played by a particular circulating cell, the monocyte. The key to chronic inflammation lies in the biology of these cells just as in acute inflammation it lies in the properties of the vascular endothelial cell and the neutrophil granulocyte.

Chronic inflammation is the basis of some of the most important diseases of man and animals. Tuberculosis, leprosy and syphilis have already been mentioned and to this list should certainly be added rheumatoid arthritis, Crohn's disease and sarcoidosis as well as a variety of tropical diseases. Some industrial diseases like pneumoconiosis are also important examples. Inflammatory granulomas are characterised by massive infiltration with monocytes and their derivatives, and often by widespread death of host tissue with the formation of cavities or abscesses as in tuberculosis. Such destruction may be followed by permanent crippling as in rheumatoid arthritis in which articular cartilage is irreversibly damaged or by replacement with fibrous tissue as in silicosis.

At first sight these chronic inflammatory diseases affecting different organs, due to different and sometimes unknown causes and following different courses have nothing in common except their prolonged duration. In fact, however, the underlying pathological mechanisms are similar.

The best starting point to understand chronic inflammation and inflammatory granulomas is the monocyte and its derivative the macrophage. The monocyte comes from a precursor cell in the bone marrow, the promonocyte, and circulates in the blood. The trio of promonocyte, monocyte and macrophage makes up the mononuclear phagocyte system (p. 21). An individual monocyte does not remain long in the circulation before migrating into the tissues. It does this even when there is no inflammation but the process is enormously accelerated after local injury. Once in the tissues it enlarges and develops and becomes known as a macrophage, a name coined by Metchnikoff in the 1890s. The word means 'big eater' and refers equally well to the size of the cell, to its great capacity for phagocytosis and the large particles which it can engulf within its cytoplasm. In invertebrates it is the haematocyte, the equivalent of the macrophage, which acts as almost the sole defence against irritant particles. It does so by phagocytosis followed by digestion of the particle within the cytoplasm and it is precisely this programme which is followed by the mammalian macrophage in chronic inflammation. Chronic inflammation and the dominant role of the macrophage can therefore be viewed as an important survivor of an early phylogenetic era. The advantage of the macrophage over the other blood phagocytes, i.e. granulocytes, is its capacity to ingest bacteria and particles too large for the cells of the granulocyte series. Its other relevant property is the capacity to survive for days, weeks or months while within its cytoplasm lie bacteria, sometimes alive and even dividing. The toughness of the macrophage is due partly to its ability to resynthesise the enzymes and intracellular structures lost during phagocytosis and digestion, a property which granulocytes do not possess. It is these masses of macrophages, many containing endocytosed bacteria or other irritant particles and capable of surviving this experience, which make up the bulk of chronic inflammatory granulomas. The retention by macrophages of irritants is an obvious example of symbiosis and chronic inflammation is a phylogenetically old technique for stabilising a symbiotic relationship.

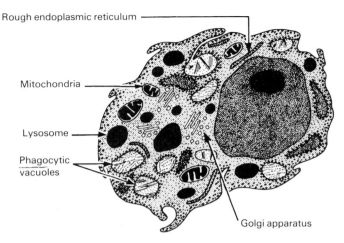

Fig. 18.1 Macrophage.

The cellular biology of the macrophage (Fig. 18.1) makes it particularly suitable to cope with alien particles which are especially difficult to kill or digest. Its wide expanse of cell membrane (plasmalemma) and active pseudopod formation facilitate pinocytosis and phagocytosis. The abundance of membrane favours the formation of intracellular phagocytic vesicles (phagosomes). The cell contains a large number and variety of lysosomes which fuse readily with the phagosomes to form secondary lysosomes in which bacteria are killed and digested. There is sufficient endoplasmic reticulum to resynthesise the lysosomal enzymes. Within the cytoplasm exist bactericidal systems which are usually effective if not fully understood (p. 23). The cell is very hardy, capable of both division and of long life and can proceed with phagocytosis and intracellular digestion under conditions of low oxygen tension. It is able to respond to information passed to it from T lymphocytes by lymphokines (p. 33) which makes it even more effective. The effect of these chemical messages is to enlarge the cell and increase its ability to divide (stimulation) and to enhance its bactericidal capacity (activation). If unable to kill a micro-organism it can at least sequester it and thus prevent unimpeded spread. The macrophage destroys micro-organisms and tissues impartially and is an effective scavenger. Its ubiquitous and versatile nature is attested by the variety of names it has acquired in special situations, e.g. graft rejection cells (in rejecting skin grafts), Aschoff cells (in rheumatic fever), heart failure cells (in the lung during cardiac failure), or compound granular corpuscles (in damaged brain).

Even trivial short-lived injury may lead to the migration of monocytes into the tissues but they persist there only if the irritant is not eliminated. Chronic inflammation is therefore caused by stimuli which while unable to destroy the host quickly cannot themselves be easily dealt with. Large bacteria of complex chemical composition, destructive but lacking maximal toxicity are the ideal pathogens for inducing such lesions.

The reason why such bacteria, e.g. tubercle bacilli are killed with such difficulty is not known. It may be that the bacilli prevent the fusion of lysosomes with the phagocytic vacuole in which they are contained. Some parasites which cause chronic inflammation become coated with host antigens once inside its body. These 'wolves in sheep's clothing' must become as impervious to attack as the host's own cells. In other cases the ingested organisms may simply be insusceptible to the macrophage's armory of bactericidal mechanisms or alternatively be shielded from them by sequestration in inaccessible parts of the cytoplasm. Even when dead the bacteria may leave indigestible chemical residues (usually the cell wall) which because they are phagocytosed, demand a local presence of macrophages which thus constitute a focus of chronic inflammation.

The peculiar marriage of indestructible bacteria or other irritants with a macrophage reaction is preceded by an initial efflux of neutrophil granulocytes, but these are quickly and permanently replaced by macrophages. It seems likely that certain types of infection or injury activate factors in serum particularly chemotactic to monocytes. The cells emigrate from blood vessels in the same way as polymorphs by inserting pseudopodia through the inter-endothelial junctions.

Once a collection of monocyte-derived macrophages is in the tissues in contact with the stubborn irritant, the host's survival demands that the macrophage accumulations persist as long as the irritant remains. In practice this accumulation is maintained in three ways. The first is by sustained migration from the circulation, balanced if the granuloma is of constant size, by a corresponding loss of cells by death or drainage to lymph nodes. The continued emigration is presumably due to the prolonged operation of factors chemotactic for monocytes. It is accompanied by some augmented release of monocytes from the bone marrow and factors have been identified in serum which act on the marrow to stimulate monocyte production (p. 97). An exaggerated response in the shape of a monocytosis is seldom seen.

The second mechanism for maintaining a macrophage population in granulomas is by mitotic division of the cells. Monocytes enlarge and tend to divide once, soon after leaving the circulation. Having settled down, they may undergo one or two further divisions but seldom more, before dying or retiring. This division is probably triggered by the local release of mitogenic compounds derived from other macrophages or other types of cell. Analysis of the chromosomes of the proliferating macrophages reveals numerous abnormalities likely to limit their viability. It is this which probably restricts the number of successful mitoses that they can achieve.

The third strategy which has evolved is the immobilisation of macrophages at the site of inflammation so that they rarely die and rarely divide. As a result a stable population of storage cells is created which is dependent for its existence neither on recruitment from the circulation nor on mitotic proliferation.

In practice granulomas fall into two categories, those with much continued emigration and division, known as high turnover granulomas, and those with a stable population of longlived macrophages, known as low-turnover granulomas (Fig. 18.2). Bacterial or fungal infections or inflammation due to irritants toxic to macrophages produce high turnover reactions. Irritants of low toxicity to macrophages, e.g. carbon particles, cause low turnover lesions.

By no means all the cells in an area of chronic inflammation have the appearance of macrophages. Some may be epithelioid cells, particularly numerous in tuberculosis and sarcoidosis, with foamy interlocking cytoplasm. These are macrophage derivatives, the cytoplasm of which seems specialised for secretion rather than phagocytosis. Epithelioid cells have only one tenth the phagocytic activity of macrophages but much more endoplasmic reticulum, Golgi apparatus, plasmalemma and exocytotic activity (Fig. 18.3). They seem

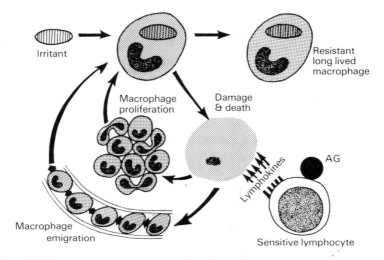

Fig. 18.2 Macrophage turnover in chronic inflammation.

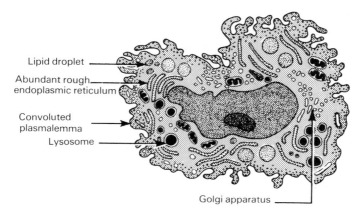

Lipid droplet

Abundant rough endoplasmic reticulum

Convoluted plasmalemma

Lysosome

Golgi apparatus

Fig. 18.3 Epithelioid cell.

particularly adapted for the extracellular secretion of lysosomal enzymes and other cytoplasmic proteins such as lysozyme which is also a property of macrophages in general. Epithelioid cells arise from macrophages or monocytes by a special kind of maturation. The maturation takes a few days to develop and is retarded if the parent macrophage undertakes phagocytosis, especially of indigestible particles. Epithelioid cells have a life of 1 to 3 weeks and when they divide produce daughter cells with the features of young macrophages. The presence of large numbers of epithelioid cells in diseases such as tuberculosis is probably due to the presence of macrophages which are immobilised but shielded from the necessity to phagocytose bacilli by a barrier of non-epithelioid macrophages. In other diseases rich in epithelioid cells, such as sarcoidosis, their presence may be due to lack of indigestible particles so that without having to undertake phagocytosis and digestion, macrophages have the leisure to undergo epithelioid maturation.

Multinucleate giant cells are another feature of granulomas. They are formed by fusion of macrophages (Fig. 18.4) and are seen in chronic inflammation whenever fresh monocytes are in constant supply as in tuberculosis. Formation of multinucleate giant cells (macrophage polykaryons) seems to depend upon intimate contact of freshly migrated monocytes simultaneously with other monocytes or macrophages, and with material demanding endocytosis. This material may be particulate, e.g. bacteria or foreign bodies, or soluble, e.g. protein-rich exudate. It seems likely that a combination of high cell density and simultaneous endocytosis of the same material by two or more macrophages is the fusion stimulus in giant cell formation (Fig.

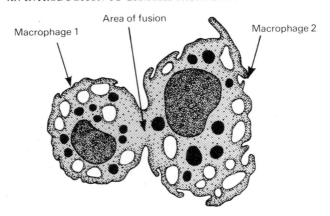

Fig. 18.4 Macrophages fusing to form multinucleate giant cells.

18.5). Classical pathology recognises foreign body and Langhans types of giant cells but the electron microscope shows the latter to be merely a more highly organised development of the former. Indeed, interference with movement of intracellular organelles by dosage with colchicine prevents the conversion of foreign body cells to Langhans' cells.

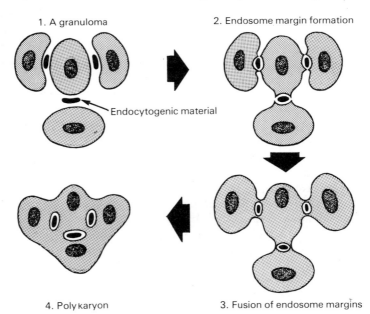

Fig. 18.5 The fusion of macrophages to form inflammatory giant cells as a result of simultaneous endocytosis of particles or colloids.

Fate	Cause
Death	Phagocytosis of toxic material
Migration from site	Disappearance of inflammatory stimulus
Division	(1) Entry into inflamed tissues (2) Exposure to mitogens
Conversion to long-lived form	Phagocytosis of non-toxic, indigestible material
Conversion to epithelioid cell	(1) Immobilisation without phagocytic activity (2) Immobilisation after successful phagocytic activity
Conversion to giant cell (macrophage polykaryon)	Co-existence of effete and young macrophages in close proximity, with simultaneous endocytosis.

Fig. 18.6 Fate of inflammatory macrophage.

Once the multinucleate cells are formed they grow by the additional fusion of macrophages. They also behave like other polykaryons in biology in that they undergo synchronous or nearly synchronous entry of nuclei into the mitotic cycle. In macrophage polykaryons this usually ends in pooling of chromosomes, many of which are defective and the resultant formation of polyploid cells of very limited life span. Thus the division of macrophages which could have ended in uncontrolled growth is neatly curtailed. Figure 18.6 shows the various fates that can befall the inflammatory macrophage.

Other cell types are also present in chronic inflammation, in

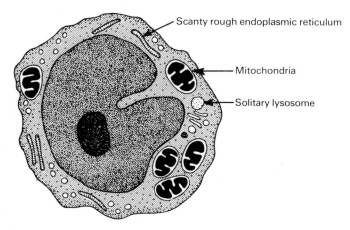

Scanty rough endoplasmic reticulum

Mitochondria

Solitary lysosome

Fig. 18.7 Small lymphocyte.

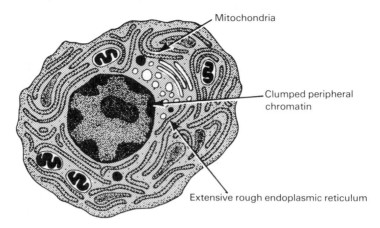

Fig. 18.8 Plasma cell.

particular lymphocytes (both T and B cells; Fig 18.7), plasma cells (Fig. 18.8) eosinophils and fibroblasts. The presence of lymphoid cells indicates some form of immunological activity and plasma cells mean that immunoglobulin is being formed. There is a close relationship between lymphocytes and macrophages since the former are able to increase the activity of the latter by the secretion of chemical substances known as lymphokines or of a material called transfer factor. This interaction seems to occur when cell-mediated immunity or hypersensitivity is present (p. 33). Under these circumstances sensitised or immune lymphocytes in contact with the appropriate antigen will instruct macrophages to migrate to the inflamed area, i.e. the site of antigen deposition and there to accumulate, die and divide. In some diseases the granulomatous reaction (Fig. 18.9) appears to depend entirely upon cell-mediated immunity, e.g. in experimental inflammation provoked by schistosome eggs. In general there are close links between granulomatous inflammation and cell-mediated immunity and the two phenomena are the main characteristics of diseases such as tuberculosis and leprosy. In tuberculosis, lymphocyte-mediated immune responses play a completely dual role in that they probably aggravate the inflammatory reaction and cause local tissue necrosis (caseation) at the centre of the tubercle while also stimulating the macrophages to ingest and destroy the tubercle bacilli. Both facets of the immune response develop progressively in adult life so that childhood tuberculosis tends to be less destructive and also less localised than the adult disease.

In diseases such as tuberculosis and leprosy the only defence of the host is the ability of the macrophage to phagocytose and kill the bacilli.

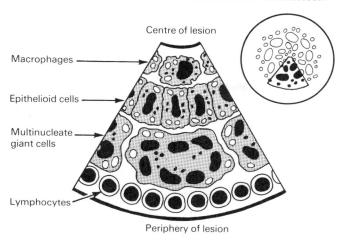

Centre of lesion

Macrophages

Epithelioid cells

Multinucleate giant cells

Lymphocytes

Periphery of lesion

Fig. 18.9 Architecture of a chronic inflammatory granuloma.

However, we have the advantage over invertebrates in which a similar system operates, in that the macrophages are rendered more efficient by the development of lymphocyte-mediated immunity. Unfortunately, as already mentioned this exaggerated response may do as much damage to the host as to the invading micro-organism. Indeed much or most of the damage in tuberculosis and leprosy is the result of the erosive action of the digestive enzymes of the lysosomes within macrophages. This is even more evident in granulomas such as rheumatoid arthritis or sarcoidosis where intensive research has failed to identify such an invader and only the infiltrating inflammatory cells can be blamed. It is widely believed that these macrophages too are reacting to an immunological stimulus which may be an exogenous agent, as yet unidentified or a component of the patient's own tissue (p. 54). A number of other diseases are suspected to have a similar origin. Although lymphocytes may conceivably damage tissue cells by direct action it is more likely that they usually kill by instructing macrophages to do so. These separate but inter-reacting cell types are set out in Figure 18.10.

Cell-mediated hypersensitivity is then specially associated with chronic inflammation. When hypersensitivity is absent the tissue destruction and continued emigration and division of macrophages in chronic inflammation is most likely to be due to leakage and secretion of lysosomal enzymes and other cytoplasmic irritants from the macrophage into the tissues. This escape of damaging substances is sometimes accelerated by phagocytic activity. It is the most likely

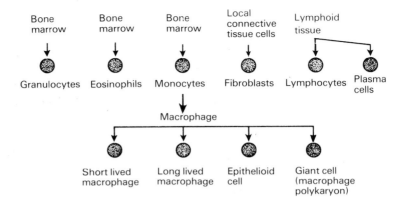

Fig. 18.10 The cells of inflammation.

explanation of diseases such as silicosis which are associated with uptake by macrophages over long periods of time of material which is both indigestible and toxic but not obviously immunogenic. Macrophages undertaking phagocytosis also release a substance which stimulates fibroblasts to divide and to make collagen, so the connection between chronic irritation, granuloma formation, tissue destruction and scarring, especially prominent in silicosis, seems to be complete (Fig. 18.11).

One other aspect of chronic irritation is of importance. This is the permanent increase in secretion of viscid mucus which occurs from the epithelial cells lining the bronchial tree when there is prolonged inhalation of irritants. A chronic excess of bronchial mucus is the pathological basis of chronic bronchitis, a disease which killed 22 000 people in England in 1977. Of the inhaled irritants, cigarette smoke is probably the most important but atmospheric pollutants such as sulphur dioxide and smoke are also heavily implicated. Ironically, but

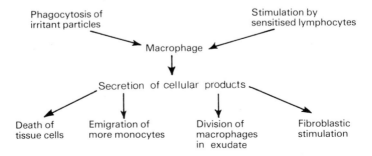

Fig. 18.11 The central role of the macrophage in chronic inflammation.

predictably, chronic bronchitis, which was once called the 'English disease', is now a major cause of death in Hong Kong, Tokyo and São Paulo.

As pointed out earlier (p. 10) secretion of respiratory mucus is a useful defence, especially against inhaled bacteria. It is predictable that some means of increasing this secretion in the face of repeated irritation would have evolved by natural selection and the respiratory epithelium of patients with chronic bronchitis show evidence of enlargement of the mucus secretory glands and increase in their number. Unfortunately this prolonged over-stimulation causes the air passages to become clogged with sticky secretion. As a result, instead of being preserved, lung function is eventually irretrievably damaged.

Bibliography

Boros D L 1978 Granulomatous inflammation. Progress in Allergy 24: 183

Chambers T J 1978 Multinucleate giant cells. Journal of Pathology 126: 125

Kilburne K H (ed) 1974 Pulmonary reactions to organic materials. Annals of the New York Academy of Sciences, vol. 227

Spector W G 1974 The macrophage: its origins and role in pathology. In: Ioachim H L (ed) Pathobiology Annual. Appleton Century Crofts, New York

Van Furth R (ed) 1975 Mononuclear Phagocytes in immunity, infection and pathology Blackwell, Oxford

Weissmann G, Samuelsson B, Paoletti R (eds) 1979 Advances in inflammation research vol 1. Raven Press, New York

19

Atheroma

Atheroma (from a Greek word meaning porridge) is an arterial disease the complications of which kill more people in the Western world than any other disease, including cancer. Atheroma can affect all arteries above 2 mm in diameter but is most important in the aorta, cerebral, coronary, mesenteric and femoral arteries. It is the major cause of heart attacks and strokes, it is an important factor in senility and it is the major complication in diabetes.

To understand atheroma it is first necessary to recapitulate the normal architecture of the large and medium sized arteries (Fig. 19.1). The lumen of these vessels is lined by a single layer of flattened cells, the endothelium. They form the inner boundary of a narrow layer called the intima whose outer boundary is the internal elastic lamina. Normally the intima is composed of a few smooth muscle cells, collagen fibres and glucosaminoglycans (proteoglycans, mucopolysaccharides, ground substance). The internal elastic lamina is an incomplete layer of fibres of elastin, a protein secreted by the arterial smooth muscle cells. Beyond the internal elastic lamina is the media, which is composed of smooth muscle cells separated by small amounts of collagen, elastin and glucosaminoglycans. There are no fibroblasts in the intima or media of mammalian arteries. The adventitia is the outermost coat and is separated from the media by a loose elastin barrier, the external elastic lamina. The adventitia consists of fibroblasts, collagen and glucosaminoglycans and in larger arteries is supplied by small blood vessels, the vasa vasorum.

The essential pathological change which distinguishes an atheromatous artery from a normal vessel is the accumulation in the intima of collagen and of the lipid material which has given the disease its name. This fat consists mainly of cholesterol and cholesterol esters and triglycerides. It is associated with large amounts of collagen and glucosaminoglycans and with greatly increased numbers of smooth muscle cells. Some of the fat is in the cytoplasm of these cells, some within macrophages and some is extracellular. The combination of lipid, fibrous tissue and cells has led to the use of the term atheroscler-

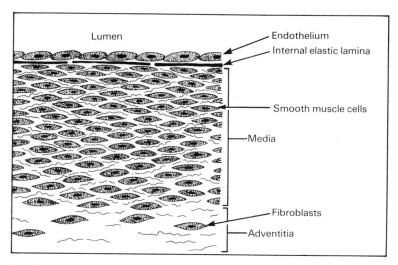

Fig. 19.1 Cross section of normal coronary artery

osis as a synonym for atheroma, although Scottish pathologists have objected to it on the etymological ground that it means 'hard porridge', a concept which they find unacceptable.

The fat and fibrous tissue accumulate as localised plaques which project into the lumen of the vessel and significantly narrow it in the smaller arteries (Fig. 19.2). When fibrous tissue is prominent it appears as a white nodule or thickening but beneath it, deeper in the intima, lies a mass of yellow lipid. Sometimes atheroma is present

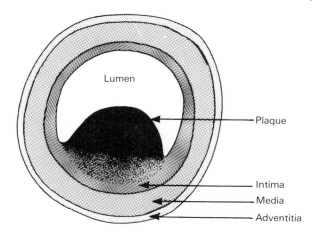

Fig. 19.2 Partial blockage of a coronary or cerebral artery by atheroma.

simply as fatty streaks in the intima. These consist initially of lipid within the cytoplasm of smooth muscle cells. Fatty streaks are seen in the aortas of even young children and it is widely believed that they represent the earliest lesions of atheroma. However, it is known that such deposits may disappear as well as progress and it is by no means certain that progression to a fibrous fatty plaque is their usual fate.

In advanced cases of atheroma, the fibro-fatty plaque becomes subject to a variety of complications including deposition of calcium salts, bleeding into the plaque, necrosis of its constituent tissues, ulceration of the bulging intimal surface or even rupture of the plaque itself.

Almost all middle-aged or elderly people dying of other causes or diseases show atheroma, certainly of the aorta, probably of the coronary, femoral and cerebral arteries. In such cases there is often no evidence that atheroma caused any symptoms or contributed to death. Of all individuals dying, however, almost half do so as a result of the complications of atheroma.

Of these complications, thrombosis is the most important. Thrombosis is discussed elsewhere (p. 140) but it consists essentially of the agglutination of blood platelets on a vascular surface. This forms a platelet mass which projects into the lumen and causes ordinary blood clot to form which in turn acts as a stimulus for more platelet agglutination and so on. Thrombus formation on an aortic plaque of atheroma is commonplace and unimportant, since the lumen of the vessel is too wide for the blood flow to be obstructed by the flattened thrombus. In the coronary or cerebral vessels, however, a thrombus builds up rapidly to occlude the lumen totally. The result is an infarct, i.e. death of an area of tissue due to sudden and complete deprivation of arterial blood supply (p. 150). Clinically this will be manifest as a heart attack or a stroke, the two commonest causes of death in all societies which have eradicated malnutrition and infections as competitors for this title. As between heart attacks or strokes, i.e. cardiac or cerebral infarcts, the heart is the more important, partly because it kills more people but mainly because of its tendency to appear early in middle age or even younger. Cardiac infarction together with less sudden manifestations of reduced coronary blood flow, e.g. heart failure or angina pectoris, constitute the cluster of maladies known as ischaemic heart disease (IHD). Strokes, too, however, sometimes occur in youngish and active middle-aged people, with resultant physical and mental disability. In terms of total numbers, however, most cardiac and cerebral infarcts occur in elderly people. They are therefore the most common termination of the ageing process of which atheroma is the most prominent or at least the most easily identified feature.

Thrombosis is not the only serious complication. Atheroma also causes aneurysms of the aorta due to local dilatation, as a result of destruction of normal constituents especially elastic fibres. Aneurysms may rupture and cause death but if diagnosed earlier the affected aortic segment can be excised and replaced by a tube of woven synthetic fibres. A form of aneurysm not due to atheroma but also prevalent in middle-aged or elderly males is dissecting aneurysm of the aorta. This is due to degeneration of the media often associated with hypertension. Blood appears in the medial coat either by a crack in the intima or from a ruptured vasa vasorum. The blood finds its way between the middle and outer thirds of the media and dissects them apart. Another risk in atheroma is that a portion of fatty necrotic tissue may soften enough to become detached and be swept to another part of the arterial tree where it may block a vessel and cause an infarct. A similar effect may arise from the dislodgement of an adherent thrombus. The process of detachment, circulation and lodgement is known as embolus formation and is an important pathological mechanism (p. 150). Atheroma may affect the valves of the heart, causing interference with the opening and closing of the valves and leading to heart failure.

The causes of atheroma and the mechanisms whereby they establish the disease are fascinating subjects made more complex by the possibility that some complications, especially coronary artery thrombosis may have their own causal factors. As diseases are unravelled, starting from total ignorance and progressing to understanding and prevention or cure, medical history shows that comprehension comes in a predictable sequence. At first there develops a correlation of disease with particular circumstances at the purely anecdotal level. This stimulates properly conducted statistical and epidemiological studies. As these techniques become progressively refined so the correlations become more precise. At this stage it is possible to make definite statements, e.g. cigarette smoking is closely associated with lung cancer. Having identified an associated circumstance attempts are now made to show that the factor actually causes the disease. This may be done in laboratory animals or even in human volunteers. If this hurdle is jumped all that remains is to demonstrate that removing or neutralising the factor prevents or cures the disease.

This laborious sequence has been pursued with total success in almost all of the infections which used to kill men in their thousands or millions. It has been achieved in tuberculosis, syphilis, diphtheria, plague and smallpox. It has almost been achieved in cancer of the lung since although the cancer-inducing agent in cigarettes has yet to be identified, there is no doubt that abstinence from cigarette smoking reduces the risk of developing cancer of the lung to negligible levels.

In the case of atheroma it has long been obvious that advancing age and high standards of nutrition are associated factors. In Western countries, in people over 60 yrs old atheroma is always demonstrable and usually extensive so that in this special context disease can be said to be the norm. The exceptions are provided mainly by those suffering from prolonged malnutrition or wasting diseases. Here regression of lesions may have occurred prior to death if the calcification, ulceration etc. have not progressed too far.

Because of the normality of atheroma above a certain age, attention has been directed to factors inducing atheroma at an unusually early age or to a particularly severe degree. Some diseases, such as diabetes mellitus or myxoedema (lack of thyroid hormone) have long had this reputation. There is a correlation between obesity and early developing atheroma. At this stage it should be pointed out that evidence of premature or unduly severe atheroma comes mainly from the onset of the complications of atheroma especially cardiac infarcts. This undoubtedly introduces the possibility that quite separate agents may be operative, but as we shall see there is remarkably good correspondence between atheroma-producing factors and heart attacks. Another important condition that has a high correlation with premature atheroma and cardiac infarction is hypertension, i.e. abnormally high arterial blood pressure. If the hypertension is confined to the pulmonary circulation (a relatively rare circumstance) atheroma develops only in the pulmonary artery, wheareas the arteries of the lung normally escape atheromatous change. Familial tendencies have been shown to be important in premature atheroma and cardiac infarction. The sex of the individual is important since at the age of 45 years heart attacks are seven times more common in men than in women. In older age groups the difference is much less striking. Cigarette smoking has a statistically significant association with heart attacks and in matched controls has been shown to be associated with larger atheromatous deposits. Occupation appears to be related to cardiac infarction since those in sedentary jobs appear to be more at risk than those obliged to exercise. Psychological stress is also a risk factor although one which is not easy to assess. Sedentary hobbies carry a higher statistical risk than vigorous ones such as gardening. Emotional disturbances or depression due to bereavement, frustrated ambition or fear of poverty seem to be risk factors, at least at the anecdotal level. Diet is an important factor since total daily calories and intake of saturated animal fats have highly significant statistical correlations with cardiac infarction. A diet rich in starch and sugar has a similar effect.

It is apparent that we have a formidable list of circumstances, each of which has a statistical correlation with premature or unduly severe atheroma and cardiac infarction. The list embraces age, male gender, diabetes, high blood pressure, inherited tendencies, cigarette smoking, sedentary jobs and habits, obesity, diet and psychological trauma. It is obvious therefore that there is no single cause of atheroma or of its complications, cardiac infarction and ischaemic heart disease. On the other hand it seems unlikely that no general mechanisms exist through which these diverse factors work.

In fact three such general pathways probably operate. The first is elevation of the low density lipoproteins (LDL) of the plasma. Cholesterol and triglyceride is carried in the blood combined with proteins as lipoproteins. The higher the content of lipid in the molecule the lower the density of the lipoprotein since lipid is lighter, i.e. less dense, than protein. There is a very clear cut correlation between the level of LDL in the blood and the incidence of ischaemic heart disease. In practice, LDL is measured by estimation of blood cholesterol and triglyceride since these are the main lipid constitutents of LDL. Blood cholesterol increases steadily with age, in males rising by 25 per cent between the ages of 20 and 50 years. It also correlates well with obesity. Women have lower levels in the younger age groups and tend to approximate to male concentrations after the menopause. Diabetes mellitus and hypothyroidism both of which predispose to atheroma are associated with high cholesterol levels. There are several inherited conditions in which there is an excess of various types of lipoproteins in the blood (familial hyperlipidaemia). Such families may have a greatly increased risk of premature cardiac infarction. In two types, (IIa and IIb) half the sufferers have ischaemic heart disease by the age of 49 years (see Ch. 15).

Diets rich in saturated animal fat raise blood cholestarol and diets in which animal fat is replaced by polyunsaturated vegetable fat, lower it. A starchy diet raises the blood triglyceride level.

It is apparent therefore that the effects of male gender, age, diabetes, obesity, diet and familial tendencies can all be attributed to high levels or circulating cholesterol and triglyceride present as LDL. This seems to account for some of the factors implicated in atheroma, but if so, lowering the plasma LDL concentration should reduce the incidence of cardiac infarcts compared with matched controls. This experiment is difficult to perform because of the long time scale required, but it can be monitored by the blood lipid levels and people can be found who are prepared to give up flavoursome animal fat for possibly more healthy diets. In the USA, Great Britain, Finland, Norway and the Netherlands this experiment has been conducted and the incidence of atheroma and its complications, i.e. cardiac and cerebral infarction reduced by as much as 30 per cent.

More recently, attention has been focussed on the role of low levels of high density lipoproteins (HDL). These have a high proportion of protein to cholesterol in their molecule. In several epidemiological studies a good correlation has been found between low levels of circulating HDL and the incidence of atheromatous coronary artery disease. On the other hand whereas familial diseases in which LDL are raised are associated with a very high risk of ischaemic heart disease, the same is not true of similar rare diseases in which HDL levels are abnormally low. It may be that low amounts of circulating HDL is a risk factor only when the tendency for LDL to accumulate in arterial walls is already present. The HDL could, for example, bind cholesterol which would otherwise accumulate in arterial walls, or compete with LDL for binding sites in the vessel wall. It may also be that the real significance of high HDL levels is that they indicate adequate amounts of the enzyme lipoprotein lipase (LPL) since the two seem to be positively related. It is of interest also, that another protective factor against coronary heart disease, regular physical exercise, has a similar direct relationship with LPL levels in the blood.

This situation is satisfying as far as it goes but leaves many factors unexplained, notably hypertension and cigarette smoking which do not correlate with blood lipids. The effect of high blood pressure and of cigarettes is probably to damage the arterial wall and to increase its permeability to blood constituents, including lipoprotein (Fig. 19.3). Mechanical damage in conjunction with high blood cholestrol has long been known to cause atheroma when experimentally induced in animals. More specifically if the lining endothelium of a major artery is stripped off by passage of a rubber tube which is inflated and then withdrawn, atheromatous plaques develop at the site of injury but not elsewhere. With regard to cigarettes there are several ways in which they could damage the integrity of vessels, e.g. by causing arterial spasm or by leading to sustained high levels of carbon monoxide. Psychological stress and frustration might cause spasmodic rises in blood pressure, with ensuing arterial damage.

The third general pathway is agglutination of platelets. If this were to occur on undamaged endothelium, the release of lysosomal enzymes from the platelets might destroy the integrity of the endothelium and allow lipoproteins to enter the intima. Many of the factors which cause a rise in LDL also induce platelets to agglutinate, due perhaps to the high levels of circulating free fatty acids which are associated with

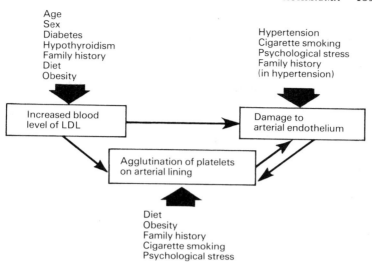

Fig. 19.3 Inter-relationship of blood lipid, arterial damage and platelet aggregation in the causation of atheroma.

elevated concentrations in the blood of LDL. In addition, disturbances which strain the endothelial lining of vessel walls, e.g. adrenalin secretion or cigarette smoking, may also make platelets more liable to clump.

We are left then with three basic mechanisms for the induction of atheroma, high levels of circulating lipoprotein, damage to the arterial endothelium and platelet agglutination. These three mechanisms may act alone or in deadly cooperation. In other words the characteristic lesions of atheroma result from increased entry of LDL into the vessel wall due to high levels of circulating LDL alone or in combination with local agglutination of platelets or with increased permeability of the endothelial barrier which separates the intima from the blood. High blood pressure could increase filtration of LDL into the artery and also damage the endothelium and make it allow the entry of LDL in abnormal amounts. The high incidence of atheroma and ischaemic heart disease in youngish black women in the USA appears to be due almost entirely to hypertension. It should be explained that the intima normally receives its nutriment by diffusion from the blood so that increased entry of LDL can be regarded as an exaggeration of a physiological process.

There is no doubt that interference with the intergrity of the lining endothelium allows atheromatous plaques to form in the intima (Fig. 19.4). There is also no doubt that these plaques contain LDL identical

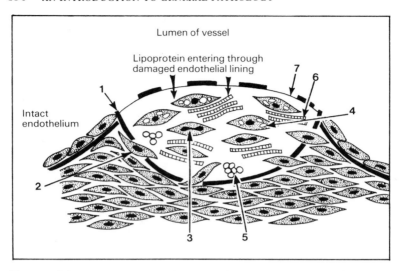

Fig. 19.4 Atheromatous plaque: 1 Fragmented internal elastic lumen; 2. Smooth muscle cells migrating into intima; 3. Dividing smooth muscle cells; 4. Lipid in smooth muscle cells; 5. Extra cellular lipid; 6. Newly synthesised collagen; 7. Naked subendothelial surface.

with that found in plasma. They also contain fibrinogen but other plasma proteins are generally not demonstrable. The retention of LDL and fibrinogen is due partly to their high molecular weight, and partly to selective precipitation with charged calcium-rich sulphated glucosaminoglycans which are also present in the plaques. Since fibrinogen is an important constituent of atheromatous lesions it is of interest that the erythrocyte sedimentation rate (p. 103) which largely depends on blood fibrinogen concentration has a linear correlation with overall mortality in men over 55 years old.

It used to be thought that the fibrosis in atheromatous vessels was excited by the irritant action of the lipid accumulation as if it were an example of chronic inflammation (p. 116). Except in birds, however, there are no fibroblasts in the aortic intima, only smooth muscle cells. The origin of the fibrosis in atheroma is now much clearer following the recent discovery that the smooth muscle cells in the aortic intima can synthesise collagen and glucosaminoglycans. Equally important is the recent demonstration that platelets contain a factor which stimulates the smooth muscle cells to divide and to synthesise and secrete connective tissue constituents. Activation of smooth muscle cells by the platelet factor is accompanied by a tendency for the cells to accumulate lipid droplets, as they do in atheromatous plaques (Fig. 19.5). Another interesting feature of the smooth muscle proliferation

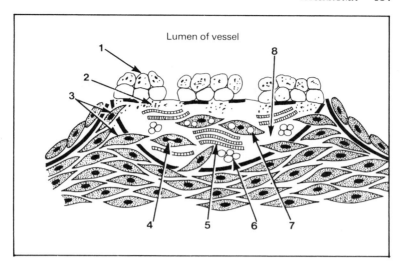

Fig. 19.5 Atheromatous plaque: 1. Adherent platelets; 2. Lysosomes discharged from platelets; 3. Migrating smooth muscle cells; 4. Dividing smooth muscle cell; 5. Newly synthesised collagen; 6. Extracellular lipid; 7. Lipid-laden smooth muscle cell; 8. Lipoprotein entering from plasma.

is that in most cases it involves only an identifiable subset of the whole cell population. This observation was made by Benditt who suggested that such 'monoclonal' proliferation should be regarded as neoplasia (p. 242). A simpler explanation is that senescence and other factors restrict the ability of the cell population to respond to stimulation so that the plaque is likely to consist of the progeny of a selected few.

The importance of the observation by Ross that platelets stimulate aortic smooth muscle cells, lies in the fact that platelet aggregation commonly occurs on sites of damaged arterial endothelium and platelet aggregation is measurably diminished by experimental diets deficient in saturated animal fats which lower the incidence of early-developing atheroma. Thus platelets are a major factor both in the lethal thrombotic complications (p. 140) and in the formation of the atheromatous plaque itself. These observations have a special interest because one of the older theories was that the atheromatous plaque consisted of a thrombus which had been incorporated into the arterial wall. The hypothesis was formulated and indeed demonstrated by the Scottish pathologist Duguid but the concept of atheroma as injury followed by proliferation can be traced to Virchow.

To make all these observations fit a simple scheme of pathogenesis it is necessary to visualise a pathway which starts with initial damage to endothelium due to age, hypertension or increased lipid entry due to high LDL (Fig. 19.6). This could lead to platelet aggregation which in turn, would cause smooth muscle cell hyperplasia and connective tissue overgrowth. With disorganisation of the intima there would be further entry and binding of lipoproteins, naturally accelerated if the circulating LDL are high. In this way a progressive failure of adaptation typical of pathology could develop.

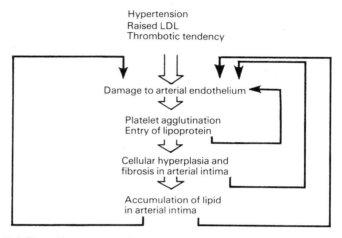

Hypertension
Raised LDL
Thrombotic tendency

Damage to arterial endothelium

Platelet agglutination
Entry of lipoprotein

Cellular hyperplasia and
fibrosis in arterial intima

Accumulation of lipid
in arterial intima

Fig. 19.6 The self-perpetuating factors in the development of atheroma.

Unlike many other important pathological processes, atheroma does not at first sight seem to be an unfortunate side effect of a survival mechanism. On the other hand, given the structure of the mammalian aorta and especially the avascular intima and the necessity to nourish it by diffusion from the blood of proteins and lipids, the disease seems inevitable. Since platelets play a major role, then atheroma is certainly a by-product of a life preserving mechanism (p. 168).

Moving from the individual to the species, atheroma can be seen as helpful in that it sets a term to the life of the members of a community who have passed the optimal age for procreation and obtaining food. Whether this can be attributed to natural selection could be hotly contested. However, if susceptibility to atheroma in middle age were genetically linked to attributes such as sexual drive, energy, intelligence and success during the procreative age span it might be selected for. Since such success is likely to be accompanied by changes in diet and life style favourable to the development of atheroma the process should proceed at an accelerating rate, a prediction which shows every sign of being fulfilled except where the life style is becoming healthier.

Bibliography

Benditt E P (ed) 1977 Atherosclerosis; a new look at the problem. American
    Journal of Pathology 86: 656
Cotton D W K (ed) 1973 Lipid metabolism and atherosclerosis. Excerpta Medica,
    Amsterdam
Lancet 1978 Editorial Lancet ii: 1291
Ross R, Glomset J A 1976 The pathogenesis of atherosclerosis. New England
    Journal of Medicine 195: 369 and 420
Tell A R, Small D M 1978 Current concepts: Plasma high density lipoprotein.
    New England Journal of Medicine 299: 1232
Vogel H G (ed) 1973 Connective tissue and ageing. Excerpta Medica, Amsterdam
Wagner W D, Clarkson T B (eds) 1974 Arterial mesenchyme and arteriosclerosis.
    Plenum, New York

20

Thrombosis

A thrombus is a solid mass or plug, formed from blood constituents in the living circulation. Thrombosis is of course the process whereby thrombi are formed. Thrombosis must be distinguished from blood clotting or coagulation which is the solidification of blood under static conditions outside the body. On the other hand it is equally important to stress that haemostasis, i.e. the arrest of haemorrhage, consists essentially of two processes, coagulation being one, the other being composed of at least some of the stages of thrombosis.

Thrombosis begins with the adhesion of platelets (Fig. 20.1) to the vessel wall and their clumping together to form a plug. This plug helps to arrest bleeding from damaged blood vessels and may thereby save our lives, but it is also the nucleus of thrombus formation which, as we have seen in the previous chapter, is frequently fatal.

Looked at with the naked eye (Fig. 20.2) a thrombus will usually be found to have taken the shape of the vessel in which it is formed and whose lumen it has blocked (an occluding thrombus) or to be more or less flattened against the wall of a larger vessel (a mural thrombus) or to be a warty excrescence on a heart valve (a vegetation). It is usually red in colour with pale areas but may be more uniformly pale. It is

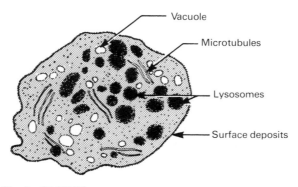

Fig. 20.1 Platelet (× 35000).

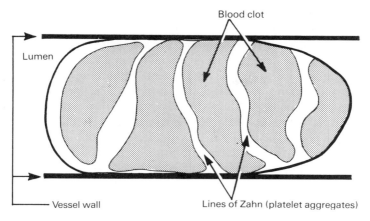

Fig. 20.2 Naked eye appearance of an occluding thrombus.

normally dry and firm and adherent to the wall of the vessel in which it has developed. If of any size it will be observed to have a striated appearance (the lines of Zahn). These striations represent the edges of the platelet masses referred to and make up most of the pale areas of the thrombus (Fig. 20.3). The spaces between the platelet clumps are filled with red corpuscles, white cells and fibrin, red cells predominating. Thus the red parts of a thrombus are very similar to ordinary blood clot in which fibrin polymerises as a network, trapping large numbers of red blood corpuscles.

Occluding thrombi form in veins and arteries and mural thrombi in the chambers of the heart and in the aorta, where they are a common sight on atheromatous plaques (p. 129). Heart valve thrombi (vegetations) form when the valve is inflamed as a result of rheumatic,

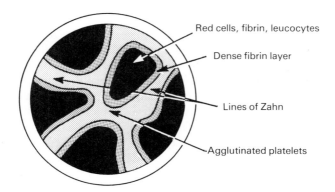

Fig. 20.3 Cross-section of thrombus.

mechanical or bacterial damage. The commonest site of venous thrombosis is the veins of the leg, deep or superficial and the commonest sites of arterial thrombosis are where atheroma is most frequent, i.e. the coronary, cerebral and femoral arteries.

The mixed nature of the constituents of thrombi is evident in sections looked at under the light microscope. The lines of Zahn are seen as pale-staining bands of virtually structureless material. In fact they are masses of platelets which have lost their cell wall, and fused to become an amorphous jelly. Lying on the surface of these bands is a narrow zone of dense strands of fibrin with a layer of white cells. The main bulk of the thrombus is occupied by blood clot which fills up the spaces between the lines of Zahn. The clot is seen to consist of masses of red cells many of which have lost their outlines, intersected by strands of fibrin and dotted with white cells present in the numbers proportionate to their concentration in blood.

The composition of thrombi is similar in all situations but the constituents vary quantitatively. In particular, venous thrombi have a higher proportion of blood clot to platelets. This is due largely to the ease with which a platelet plug can cause stasis in the slow flowing venous blood compared with fast flowing arterial blood or the blood flowing over heart valves. Thus the rheology (flow characteristics) and anatomy of veins ensure that the bulk of any venous thrombus is made up of dark red clot with only small areas of massed platelets. The platelets tend to agglutinate in vein pockets and the mass so formed grows or propagates to a size sufficient to block the blood flow and cause stasis in the vein segment back to the entry of the next distal tributary. This column of blood then clots so that retrograde spread occurs and the whole vein, commonly the femoral, may be blocked by clot (Fig. 20.4).

Venous thrombi differ in their epidemiology from those formed elsewhere. Arterial thrombi are best thought of simply as a complication of atheroma. Heart valve thrombi (vegetations) are a complication of endocarditis, i.e. inflamed heart valves. Thrombi inside the heart chambers are due to disturbances of cardiac rhythm or to cardiac infarction. Venous thrombi, however, occur usually in normal veins in patients immobilised in bed, recovering from an operation or from childbirth or suffering from heart failure. The slight tendency of the oestrogen/progesterone contraceptive pill to increase the incidence of thrombosis is seen mainly in the veins. In general, the pill causes arterial thrombosis only if arterial disease is already present.

Thrombosis anywhere occurs if one or more of three abnormalities is present. These three are disturbances in blood flow, disturbances of the surface over which the blood flows and abnormalities in the blood

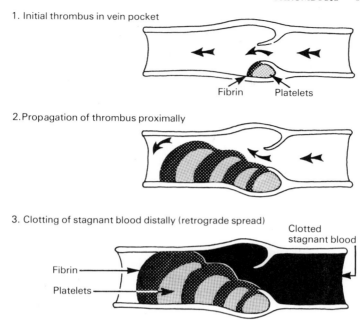

1. Initial thrombus in vein pocket

Fibrin   Platelets

2. Propagation of thrombus proximally

3. Clotting of stagnant blood distally (retrograde spread)

Clotted stagnant blood

Fibrin

Platelets

Fig. 20.4 The stages of venous thrombosis.

constituents involved in coagulation. The three make up Virchow's Triad, proposed a century ago by Virchow, the father of cellular pathology. They were based on a theoretical analysis and have stood up well to the passage of time.

The essential first step in all thrombus formation is the adhesion of platelets to the vascular surface. The electron microscope reveals this step particularly well, especially in experimentally induced thrombosis. The platelets are seen to form a craggy edifice jutting into the lumen. At first the individual platelets are intact but later lose their cellular inclusions and fuse. The point of attachment to the vessel wall is clearly shown to be penetration of one or more platelets to the subendothelial tissues, usually the basement membrane. At the luminal surface of the platelet mass is a fringed layer composed of platelets which have lost their granules and altered their shape. This layer is important because to its irregular surface is attached the dense band of fibrin and leucocytes previously mentioned (Fig. 20.5).

All the experimental data suggests that loss of integrity of the vascular endothelial lining and consequent exposure of the underlying structures of the vessel wall is the essential prerequisite for thrombus formation. In atheroma this process seems certain to occur because of

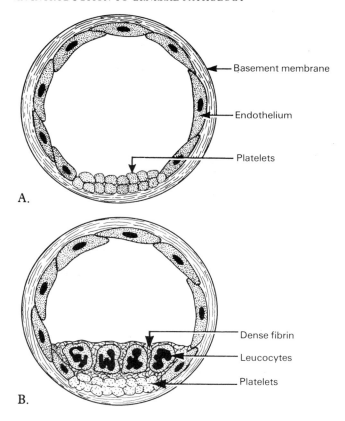

A.

Basement membrane

Endothelium

Platelets

Dense fibrin

Leucocytes

Platelets

B.

the very nature of the atheromatous plaque (p. 129). On inflamed heart valves, loss of endothelium and exposure of basement membrane is a reasonably predictable event. On damaged heart muscle, collagen could well be exposed to blood platelets as part of a general disruption of architecture. It is evident that platelets which come into contact with collagen in the endothelial basement membrane will adhere to the exposed surface and may initiate a thrombus but it is not clear why they do so. One possibility is that an enzyme, glucosyltransferase, which is present at the platelet surface, locks on to its carbohydrate substrate on the collagen molecule. The presence of this matching enzyme and substrate could be regarded as fortuitous but it is more likely to have evolved as part of the haemostatic plugging mechanism. Another possibility is that soluble products of collagen cause platelets to agglutinate when in the vicinity of collagen. This reaction can certainly be demonstrated in a test tube. In the case of atheroma it is known that the fatty material in the atheromatous plaque also can

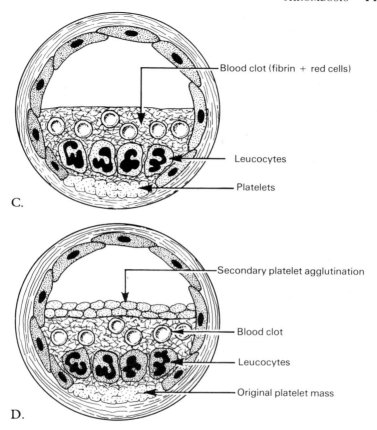

Fig. 20.5 The four stages of thrombus formation: A, Platelets stick to basement membrane; B, Dense layer of fibrin and leucocytes adhere to surface of platelets; C, Blood clot forms on surface of leucocyte/platelet layer; D, Fresh platelets agglutinate on surface of the blood clot.

cause platelets to clump together and thereby initiate a thrombus on the surface of the affected artery.

Adhesion to an exposed subendothelial surface could equally well cause thrombi to form in veins if only the inner surface of the veins could be shown to be damaged in this way. Such damage is seldom if ever demonstrable and in natural as opposed to experimental venous thrombosis, the platelet mass seems to adhere to an apparently normal endothelial surface. Evidence of preceding inflammation is hardly ever seen so any 'phlebitis' (inflammation of veins) present, comes as a sequel to the thrombosis. It is of course possible that the venous endothelium suffer invisible damage due for example to anoxia caused by sluggish blood flow.

The rather mysterious connection between endothelial cell damage, visible or invisible, and local platelet aggregation has been made much clearer by recent discoveries initiated by Vane and his colleagues. The essence of this major advance is the discovery that healthy arterial and venous endothelial cells constantly synthesise a short-lived labile substance which is the most potent known inhibitor of platelet aggregation. This remarkable compound is called prostacyclin, (often written as PGI_2, p. 65). Prostacyclin prevents platelet aggregation by increasing the concentration of cyclic AMP inside the platelets to levels which make aggregation impossible. Prostacyclin synthesis is greatly reduced in atheromatous arteries and may be reasonably presumed to be diminished after even mild damage to vascular endothelium. When this happens, the platelets in the affected vessel will be liable to agglutination by any available stimulus, e.g. collagen, or the proaggretatory thromboxane A_2, produced by the platelets themselves. Both prostacyclin and thromboxane A_2 are intermediates in the metabolism of arachidonic acid to prostglandins and illustrate the curious tendency of the members of this family to antagonise each other's biological effects. Although the advent of prostacyclin has thrown its spotlight on the vascular endothelium, there is much evidence that in venous thrombosis increased coagulability of the blood is of major importance. This hypercoagulability can sometimes be traced to lack of a particular inhibitor of a single clotting factor, e.g. factor X. That the process should nevertheless begin with platelet adhesion is explicable by the presence on the platelet surface of many factors involved in the blood-clotting mechanism. Another possibility is that the initial platelet deposition is due primarily to a local disturbance of blood flow in which the platelets become stranded like deposits on the floor of a river which is silting up. The same process could initiate platelet thrombi in arteries or segments of arteries subject to turbulent flow, as in the coronary vessels or at the origin of major branches of the aorta.

It is clear from this discussion that all three factors of Virchow's triad are still relevant to the problem of thrombosis. Endothelial damage may be the major initiating factor in arterial or endocardial thrombosis, alterations in blood constituents the major initiating factor in venous thrombosis and disturbed blood flow an important factor in all three situations. It is likely that wherever a thrombus forms all three mechanisms sooner or later play their part. They also interact, platelets suffering mechanical damage from turbulent flow and chemical damage from contact with atheroma, while endothelial surfaces may be injured by adhesion of abnormal platelets.

At this point it is worth recalling the suggestion that atheromatous plaques may be derived from mural platelet thrombi which become incorporated into the arterial intima (p. 137). It has been shown that experimentally-provoked platelet thrombi which have been incorporated into the arterial wall take up lipid from the blood in quite large amounts although no one has been able to explain why or how they do so. Finally, there is definite evidence that platelets contain a factor capable of causing the arterial smooth muscle cells to proliferate and to synthesise collagen and glucosoaminoglycans. In other words, not only may thrombosis be the most important complication of atheroma but platelet aggregation may be a major factor in initiating and aggravating it.

In contrast to these uncertainties a good deal is known about the way in which platelets build up a thrombus once they have begun to stick to the vessel wall. The essence of a platelet thrombus is the platelet adhesion-agglutination reaction in which the cells first stick together, then lose their contents and shape and finally induce blood coagulation (Fig. 20.6). The adhesion-agglutination reaction involves a contraction of the platelet and a change of shape so that it becomes a spiny sphere. This is probably due to shortening of an intracytoplasmic contractile protein (thrombasthenin) associated with entry of calcium ions. A number of substances induce this change, e.g. ADP (adenosine diphosphate), fatty acids, thrombin, adrenalin, serotonin, collagen and antigen/antibody complexes. In every case the reaction needs

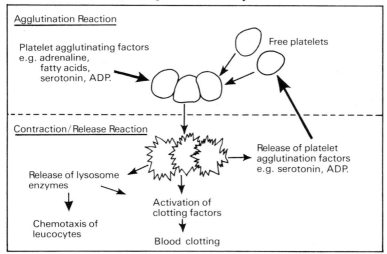

Fig. 20.6 The platelet agglutination/contraction/release reaction.

fibrinogen, indicating the close connection between platelet activation and blood clotting. Young platelets respond more readily than older cells but there is no real evidence of altered reactivity of platelets in various diseases. As might be expected, platelets have receptors for these activating substances on their surface, notably for ADP, serotonin and adrenalin. Some search has been made for a final common pathway for all these platelet agglutinating substances and a reduction in intracellular cyclic AMP has been suggested since if this change can be induced it is followed by agglutination. The prostaglandins, a family of long chain fatty acids of wide biological distribution (p. 65) may be involved here since PGI_2 inhibits platelet aggregation and also increases cyclic AMP levels and thromboxane A_2 has opposite effects. Low doses of aspirin inhibit thromboxane synthesis and higher doses inhibit PGI_2 formation. It is interesting therefore that low doses of aspirin seem to lessen the risk of thrombus formation in man.

Some of the factors listed above, which cause platelet agglutination under experimental conditions, are very much in evidence in thrombosis-promoting situations in real life. Collagen is the main constituent of basement membrane exposed to platelets when vascular endothelium is damaged; fatty acids are present in atheromatous plaques; adrenalin appears in excess in the circulation of individuals under the kind of stress that precipitates heart attacks. Antigen/antibody complexes are a major cause of damage to vessel walls and excess of clotting factors such as thrombin and fibrinogen may precipitate platelet thrombi *in vivo*.

Once the platelets have agglutinated they pass to the second stage of the reaction in which the calcium-dependent contractile protein completes its contraction. As a result there is extrusion of the granules in the platelet cytoplasm. The process is reminiscent of the reaction of polymorph leucocytes in phagocytosis and in both cases there is a burst of metabolic activity including glycolysis. The platelet granules, like those of leucocytes, are lysosomes and contain similar enzymes as well as certain factors to be mentioned later. These lysosomal enzymes can initiate many reactions and could be responsible for attraction of polymorphs to form the typical dense leucocyte layer on the platelet mass, perhaps by producing chemotatic peptides from complement (p. 28). The discharge of lysosomal enzymes coupled with the infolding of the platelet plasma membrane which occurs at this time, succeed in activating and binding the coagulation factors present in blood. In particular clotting factor X and prothrombin are converted to the active form due to the effect of platelet phospholipids known collectively as platelet factor III. Another substance released from platelets is platelet factor IV, a basic polypeptide which polymerises fibrinogen in the absence of thrombin. Thus as in the case of inflammation we see basic polypeptides released after injury (p. 64). There is also release of a factor (CPFA) which activates factor XII. These events seem very complex and somewhat tedious to relate but their importance is that the platelet release reaction does all that is necessary to induce blood clotting on the surface of the platelet mass. Indeed, it could be said to over do it, a feature which we have already seen to be common to many pathological processes. Another feature of pathological processes is self-perpetuation. In thrombosis this is demonstrated by the liberation from platelets undergoing the release reaction not only of lysosomal enzymes but also of the very factors which are most potent in initiating the agglutination/release reaction itself, namely ADP, adrenalin and serotonin. To complete matters, thrombin, which is activated by the platelet release reaction, not only causes blood to clot but also ensures completion of the release reaction itself and consolidates the platelet aggregates. Unfortunately for the patient little is left to chance.

The fate of a thrombus resembles that of an inflammatory exudate in that it may resolve or become organised, i.e. converted to connective tissue. Resolution is accomplished largely by the fibrinolytic system of the blood in which the polymerised fibrin is digested by enzyme action. Organisation occurs when fibrinolysis fails. It involves the ingrowth of fibroblasts or smooth muscle cells, laying down of collagen and proteoglycans and the formation of new endothelial-lined channels in the organised thrombus through which blood flow may be established.

Unfortunately, there is a third outcome of thrombosis, namely embolism, in which all or part of the thrombus becomes detached and enters the circulation, often with disastrous results.

Bibliography

British Medical Bulletion 1978 Thrombosis. 34: no. 2

MacIntyre D E, Pearson J O, Gordon J L 1978 Localisation and stimulation of prostacyclin production in vascular cells. Nature 271: 549

Nicolaides A N (ed) 1974 Thromboembolism. Medical and Technical Publishing Co

Poller L (ed) 1973 Recent advances in thrombosis. Churchill Livingstone, Edinburgh

21

Embolism and infarction

The real importance of thrombosis is that by blocking a blood vessel it may deprive the affected tissues of oxygenated blood. The deprivation may be partial or complete and is known as ischaemia. It may be brought about by thrombosis in the artery supplying the ischaemic part or by thrombosis elsewhere, all or some of the thrombus becoming detached, entering the blood stream and finally becoming impacted in an artery too small to allow it further passage. This latter process is known as embolism.

Although thrombi are usually thought of as the most important emboli, tumours also disseminate in this way (p. 236). Other examples are fat embolism (p. 114), air embolism and amniotic fluid embolism. Air is most likely to embolise accidentally during blood transfusion or abortion and large amounts are needed to cause death, which is due to an air lock forming in the heart. Amniotic embolism is due to debris from the amniotic cavity entering the circulation during labour and is important because it may interfere with the mother's blood clotting system.

If an embolus composed of thrombus is infected, it may at the site of impaction cause infection, inflammation or abscess formation (pyaemic abscess). The dissemination of micro-organisms by the blood stream, other than within thrombi, is not usually considered as an example of embolism, the particles being of too small a size. Genuine emboli of clumped parasites may, however, occur, as in malaria.

Another clinically important source of embolism is atheroma itself. In this instance sizeable fragments of fatty debris become dislodged from the plaque (p. 129) and are swept distally, usually only for a short distance.

Embolism and ischaemia are important and easy to understand. They are overshadowed, however, by the concept of infarction. An infarct is an area of tissue which has been acutely and completely deprived of its oxygenated blood supply and which as a result suffers tissue death. An infarct is therefore the most serious example of the general principle of ischaemia. Like many pathological terms, the word infarct is irrelevant and archaic, coming from the Latin 'infarcere' meaning to stuff (with blood). It serves to remind us of the unimportant fact that infarcts may exhibit haemorrhage due to ischaemic damage to blood vessels or show accumulation of venous blood.

Infarcts result from all the causes of arterial obstruction given above, namely local thrombosis, embolism or atheroma alone. A special case of infarction is gangrene (from a Latin and Greek word describing the actual condition). Gangrene is an infarct which has become infected by putrefactive micro-organisms. This is most likely to happen when the part, e.g. the toes of the foot, is exposed to environmental organisms or like the bowel is already inhabited by putrefactive bacteria. A particular variety is gas gangrene in which clostridia, gas-producing bacteria thriving in an oxygen-poor environment, multiply in dead tissue within the body. The dead tissue in these situations is usually the result of trauma, i.e. physical damage, and is seen in wounds and abortions.

To return to infarcts, it is useful to consider these as wounds produced by sudden loss of blood supply. Like all wounds they consist initially of dead tissue which if the patient survives will heal, i.e. become organised into new connective tissue with or without regeneration of specialised structures and cells (p. 76). In practice the latter event is rarely seen after infarction. Organisation (conversion to fibrous or scar tissue) is, however, prominent and is inevitably preceded by inflammation and phagocytosis of the dead debris by macrophages. The usual end result of an infarct is therefore a fibrous scar. Before this stage is reached, however, the microscope reveals a picture of dead tissue showing the features of cell necrosis, i.e. shrinkage (pyknosis) or disintegration (karyorrhexis) of nuclei. The cell outlines may be faintly visible or may disappear, depending on the efficiency of autolysis (auto-digestion of the cell). The dead tissue is surrounded by a zone of congested blood vessels in the surviving peripheral parenchyma. These vessels yield an inflammatory exudate (p. 69) and they and their associated structures provide the fibroblasts and blood vessels to invade and organise the infarct.

Whether or not arterial blockage produces infarction depends partly on scale (a very small interference would not be termed an infarct) and partly on alternative blood supply. Infarction of the liver is rare because there is a dual supply of oxygenated blood from the portal vein and hepatic arteries. The lung has a generous blood supply of dual origin and infarction of the lung occurs only when there is massive arterial blockage or when alternative blood supply is poor due for example to heart disease. However, since these two abnormalities

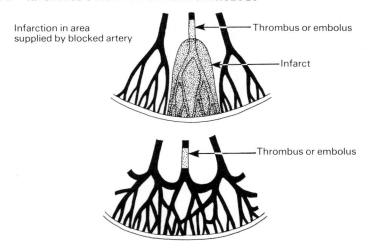

Infarction in area supplied by blocked artery

Thrombus or embolus

Infarct

Thrombus or embolus

Fig. 21.1 Prevention of infarction by collateral circulation.

frequently occur and often coexist, pulmonary infarction is a common event.

In the heart muscle there is little overlapping of the territories supplied by individual arterial branches, i.e. there is poor collateral circulation. As a result when one such branch is blocked, unless it is very small, infarction will result (Fig. 21.1). The brain has an anatomical distribution of arteries akin to the heart so that there again vascular blockage usually leads to infarction. In the kidney and spleen, arteries have a segmental distribution so infarction commonly follows arterial blockage. Some organs, e.g. retina and appendix have a single arterial supply, obstruction of which leads to infarction causing blindness and gangrenous appendicitis respectively. The limbs have a complex overlapping blood supply with many collateral branches. As a result arterial obstruction quite high up, e.g. in the femoral artery will tend to cause infarction only in a few toes. The worse the collateral circulation the larger the infarct.

Infarction of the heart muscle is the most important single cause of death in the Western world (Fig. 21.2). It is due usually to thrombosis within a branch of the coronary arteries which supply the heart with blood. The event may precipitate death immediately by causing the ventricle to cease its normal rhythmic contraction and instead to beat weakly and irregularly (fibrillation). *Spontaneous* ventricular fibrillation may lead to sudden death. If the patient survives for a few hours, a coronary thrombus may form as a secondary event, but the suggestion that coronary thrombosis is commonly the result rather than the cause

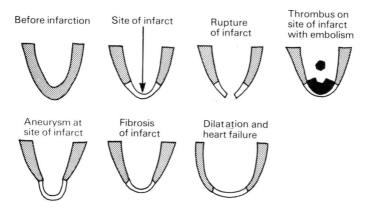

Fig. 21.2 Cardiac infarction: commonest site and complications.

of the transmural infarction shown in Figure 21.2 has no real foundation. On the other hand, diffuse myocardial necrosis known as subendocardial infarction is well known to follow subtotal coronary artery occlusion, or even dramatic reductions in myocardial perfusion as in shock (p. 113). Death from infarction may occur later due to rupture of the dead and softened heart muscle or due to cerebral embolism from thrombi formed inside the damaged heart. If a scar forms safely it may prove a poor replacement for the cardiac muscle and leave the patient partially incapacitated.

Cerebral infarcts are commonly due to embolism of the cerebral arteries and emboli may arise from atheromatous carotid arteries. Because of the extreme susceptibility of brain cells to anoxia, infarction may appear without physical obstruction of the circulation, should blood flow through the brain fall to a sufficiently low level. The vulnerability of neurones to any diminution in the supply of oxygenated blood could be predicted from the fact that although the brain makes up only about 2 per cent of the body weight it accounts for 20 per cent of the body's oxygen consumption and receives about 15 per cent of the total cardiac output.

Infarction of the lungs is usually due to an embolus from the leg veins entering the right ventricle via the inferior vena cava and the tricuspid valve and leaving via the pulmonary artery (Fig. 21.3). Such emboli may be very large and may completely block both main pulmonary arteries. However, if pulmonary circulation is faulty and collateral arterial supply not available, even smallish emboli may cause infarction.

Reproduction of infarction experimentally in liver cells shows that

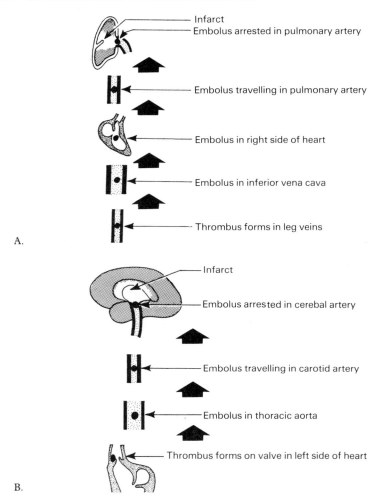

Fig. 21.3 A. Typical events in pulmonary embolism; B. Typical events in cerebral embolism.

deprivation of oxygen and enzymic substrates leads to a rapid loss of oxidative phosphorylation, and inability to oxidise Krebs cycle intermediates and a disappearance of enzyme co-factors. This loss of oxygen-dependent energy production causes a massive breakdown of ionic transport mechanisms, so that membrane potential disappears, potassium leaves the cell and sodium, water and calcium enter. In experimental systems outside the body selective replacement of oxygen, ATP, pyridine nucleotides or glycogen, may delay these events considerably. From the practical point of view, however, it is obvious that in cardiac and cerebral infarcts in living tissues, transmission of muscular and nervous impulses would be immediate casualties. In general, biosynthetic processes are more resistant to anoxia than respiration and ionic shifts but these too eventually stop.

The biochemical events of infarction are reflected in the ultrastructural changes. The mitochondria suffer at a very early stage, losing their granules, swelling and then losing their architecture. The internal membrane system of the cell quickly shows evidence of damage but the lysosomes do not suffer until hours have elapsed. The lysosomal enzymes are important in autodigestion of the cell once respiration has ceased irreversibly but probably play little part in hastening this cessation.

These biochemical events have at least one practical application in that the inability to oxidise tricarboxylic acid substrates and the general cell leakiness leads to the appearance in the circulation of enzymes involved with cell respiration whenever cell death is occurring on a large scale. The detection and measurement in the blood of enzymes such as aspartate aminotransferase or lactate dehydrogenase is a useful diagnostic test in cardiac infarction.

Cells may recover from temporary oxygen deprivation even though they suffer considerable metabolic disturbance at the time. Beyond a certain stage, however, which depends mainly on the cell type involved, the situation becomes irretrievable. Cell death is essentially an irreversible disruption of cellular respiration. Unfortunately the widespread use of mechanical ventilators has made it difficult to extend this simple concept to a generally acceptable definition of death of an individual, since by these artificial means the heart may be kept beating in the absence even of detectable life in the cerebral cortex.

Bibliography

British Medical Bulletin 1978 Thrombosis 34: no. 2
Ciba Foundation Symposium 1954 Cellular injury. Churchill, London
Davies M J, Fulton W F M, Robertson W B 1979 The relation of coronary thrombosis to ischaemic myocardial necrosis. Journal of Pathology 127: 99
Hunt A C (ed) 1972 Pathology of injury. Harvey Miller and Medcalf, Aylesbury
Morson B C (ed) 1977 Hypoxia and ischaemia. Royal College of Pathologists, London
Nicolaides A N (ed) 1974 Thromboembolism. Medical and Technical Publishing Co.

22

Cell degeneration and dysfunction

The word degeneration in pathology could be broadly defined as loss of normal structure and function, usually progressive, other than when induced by inflammation or neoplasia. Cellular degeneration is often used more simply to mean loss of normal cell structure short of cell death. Text books of pathology tend to make much play of such picturesque examples of cell degeneration as hydropic change of the kidney and fatty degeneration of the liver or heart. These appearances are of little importance except in that they indicate an underlying biochemical disturbance in the cells which compose those organs. The biochemical damage may be due to ischaemia (p. 150), to metabolic abnormalities as in diabetes, to toxic chemicals as in poisoning or to the effects of viruses or antibodies or sensitised lymphocytes (p. 42).

Cell degeneration may sometimes be merely a terminal and non-specific finding or simply an indication of widespread metabolic disturbance. On the other hand there are 4000 deaths from suicide annually in England and Wales and most of these are due to poisons whose lethal action is due to interference with cell metabolism. Alcohol abuse is one important cause of death and disease, some of the worst effects of which are due to liver damage including fatty degeneration, i.e. abnormal accumulation of lipid in hepatocytes. This is a biochemical lesion of liver cells resulting partly from a direct effect of alcohol on cellular enzyme systems. This leads to high levels of oxygen usage, increased fatty acid synthesis, decreased triglyceride synthesis and decreased secretion of lipoprotein from the liver. The other effects of alcohol are due to associated nutritional deficiencies in alcoholic subjects. These deficiencies may cause fat to accumulate by upsetting protein synthesis.

Since cell degeneration is the result of interference with cell metabolism, it obviously has close links with cell death, the latter being merely the irreversible end point of degeneration. Both are ultimately due either to a disturbance of cell enzymes, especially respiration or to disruption of cellular structures. There is also a group known as storage diseases in which certain cell constituents accumulate due to

genetically determined lack of enzymes responsible for their metabolism. These enzymes are often of lysosomal origin.

Excluding storage diseases, which are a separate problem to be
discussed later, the three main causes of cell death and dysfunction are
viruses, oxygen lack and cellular poisons, the latter including toxic
substances of bacterial, botanical, animal or synthetic origin. We have
already seen how virus infection causes cell death and degeneration (p.
16). We have also seen how in infarction severe sudden oxygen lack
leads to failure of the respiratory chain and inability to transform
energy via ATP (p. 154). This failure leads rapidly to a collapse of all
the homeostatic intracellular mechanisms governing ion transport,
membrane permeability and re-synthesis of enzymes and cell structures. Chemical poisons cause a similar progressive failure of adaptation brought about by interference with energy transforming reactions
in the cell. Where the primary attack is on something fundamental,
such as the synthesis of ATP as in dinitrophenol poisoning, or
inhibition of cytochrome oxidase by cyanide, cell death (and often
death of the patient) is the usual outcome. If the primary attack is on a
process less central to cell survival then changes short of death will
occur. In this category comes the intracellular accumulation of water
which occurs in cells in close contact with extracellular fluid, e.g.
endothelium or renal tubular epithelium when the cells are damaged.
This cellular swelling is probably due to minor disturbances in
membrane permeability or in the enzymes which control ion transport, especially the sodium pump mechanism. If there were a more
central disruption of energy transformation many other energy
dependent processes besides the sodium pump would be affected and
the cell would die.

Cyanide and dinitrophenol have been mentioned as examples of
poisons with a primary effect on the basic respiratory enzyme system.
Another classical example is fluoroacetate. This poison, once ingested,
is converted in the liver to fluorocitrate. This acts as a competitive
inhibitor of aconitate hydrolase and disrupts the oxidation of Krebs'
cycle substrates, causing cessation of respiration. The tricarboxylic
acid cycle reactions take place mainly in the mitochondria and as might
be predicted it is in the matrix of these organelles that the first
structural evidence of fluoroacetate poisoning is seen although only
after the enzyme reactions have been inhibited.

An example of a primary attack on cell structures is provided by
carbon tetrachloride which causes severe liver necrosis and fatty
degeneration if swallowed or inhaled. This substance, which is widely
used in the dry-cleaning of clothes, is harmless in itself but is
converted in the liver to free radicals which cause peroxidation of the

lipids of cell membranes, especially those forming the endoplasmic reticulum, with characteristic electron microscopic changes. This leads to disturbances of protein synthesis, probably accounting for the accumulation of neutral fat (fatty degeneration) which would otherwise have been transported by albumin or converted to lipoprotein. If membrane disruption is sufficiently serious, cell death will follow.

The two examples given, i.e. fluoroacetate and carbon tetrachloride are further illustrations of the theme that pathology is often a perversion of a homeostatic and life-preserving mechanism. Both substances are themselves harmless but are converted to toxic compounds in the liver. This is achieved by enzymes (microsomal hydroxylases) whose physiological role is to detoxify potentially harmful foods, drugs or metabolites by conjugating or hydroxylating them. It is therefore no accident that so many dangerous substances exert their worst effects on the liver and there are many other examples of conversion of chemicals to toxic forms. Of course many cellular poisons have very general effects. Cyanide has already been quoted and heavy metals such as mercury, provide another example. In mercury poisoning the sulphydryl groups of enzymes and other key substances all over the body are attacked. Even here, however, the liver's anatomical position and size make it vulnerable as it is also to toxic particulate matter such as metallic beryllium which is endocytosed by the liver's mononuclear phagocytes, known as Kupffer cells.

It can be concluded then that the visible signs of cell degeneration as defined by the light microscope are of no great importance in themselves, but that they are a significant pointer to the metabolic disturbances which occur inside cells in pathological states. It is also an appropriate reminder of the current importance of toxicology. The study of harmful substances was once a branch of forensic science. The success of modern technology, however, has greatly increased the numbers of such substances and our opportunities for encountering them. Not the least of such successes is the proliferation of new therapeutic drugs, sedatives, diuretics, antibiotics, etc. which while effective in treatment may also have harmful or even fatal actions known disarmingly as side effects. The chemistry, doses, absorption, effects and mode of action of poisons are outside the scope of this book. From the one or two examples already quoted, however, we can see how multifarious, complex and interesting are their effects on cells and how illuminating they are in exposing weak links in cellular homeostatic mechanisms.

One of the less satisfactory aspects of most accounts of cell degeneration and disruption is a tendency to concentrate on certain uncommon poisons or diseases merely because something is known of their mode of action. It is valuable therefore to examine briefly a cellular degeneration which is both clinically important and obscure, i.e. demyelination. The myelin sheath is a lipoprotein membrane that surrounds the axons or axis-cylinders of nerve fibres. In peripheral nerves it is formed by the peri-neural Schwann cells and in the central nervous system by the oligodendrocytes. The most important demyelinating disease is multiple sclerosis. It and similar diseases are characterised by fragmentation and disappearance of the myelin sheath in central nerves in the brain and spinal cord. The nerves degenerate and there is local accumulation of macrophages, lymphocytes and plasma cells followed by an increase in glial fibres. Oligodendrocytes degenerate and disappear. These disturbances result in profound abnormalities of motor and sensory function, the disease usually taking a progressive but intermittent course to total disability.

In terms of cell biology the essential element is the formation of myelin sheaths by oligodendrocytes. These cells have many extensive cytoplasmic processes which they wrap around the axon. The cell seems to make an excess of lipoprotein membrane so that it provides not only its own plasmalemma but also the myelin sheath. Multiple sclerosis may be due to auto-immunity to antigens in this lipoprotein membrane (p. 223) so that both myelin sheaths and oligodendrocytes are damaged. Certainly this effect can be demonstrated in tissue culture. Virus attack might render the lipoprotein antigenic or might infect oligodendrocytes and interfere with myelin synthesis directly. The inflammatory reaction could be secondary to the destruction of myelin or could represent an infiltration of immunogenic cells. In any case the disease seems best seen as an example of cell degeneration due to interference with the lipoprotein membrane of oligodendrocytes.

Many important diseases can be explained in terms of disordered cell biology, i.e. as examples of cell degeneration or dysfunction. In pernicious anaemia there is a grave lack of red cells due to inability to absorb the necessary vitamin B_{12} which results in turn from a lack of the gastric intrinsic factor with which dietary B_{12} combines. Intrinsic factor is a mucoprotein synthesised in the endoplasmic reticulum or Golgi apparatus. The disease is due to interference with this process which takes place in the parietal (acid secreting) cells of the stomach. The disease is characterised by disappearance of these cells together with lack of acid secretion. Acid secretion is closely linked in the cell with synthesis and secretion of intrinsic factor. Pernicious anaemia may be due to autoantibodies directed against the parietal cell itself (presumably membrane bound antigens in the endoplasmic reticulum or Golgi network) or against intrinsic factor. Other auto-immune diseases exist in which the target is the synthetic and secretory apparatus of cells in the thyroid or adrenal cortex, with predictable endocrine deficiencies.

One of the most common of all serious diseases, essential hypertension (high blood pressure of unknown cause) may be due, at least in some patients, to abnormalities in the contractile protein system of the smooth muscle cells of small arteries. This abnormality would cause narrowing of the vessels and would thereby raise the pressure within them. It is also true, however, that an increase in the number of the cells would have a similar effect.

Although essential hypertension is a disease of the greatest importance, the number and variety of postulated pathogenic mechanisms is so high that a detailed discussion is pointless. Sodium metabolism, the renin/angiotensin system, neurophysiological disturbance, catecholamines, antiduretic hormone and arginine vasopressins all have persuasive advocates.

A group of disorders known as storage diseases provide quite different examples of cell degeneration. In these maladies various substances accumulate in cells of different organs due to a genetically determined lack of the enzyme which normally catabolises the substance. Many of these diseases can now be distinguished by electron microscopic study of live liver biopsies. One example is glycogen storage disease (Von Gierkes disease) in which large amounts of glycogen accumulate in many organs due, either to lack of glucose-6-phosphatase normally found in the endoplasmic reticulum or to deficiency of one of the other enzymes involved in glycogen metabolism, some of which are in the lysosomes.

Other examples of storage diseases are the lipidoses including Gaucher's, Niemann-Pick and Tay-Sachs diseases. Here lipids accumulate in macrophages or nerve cells throughout the body due to lack of certain lysosomal enzymes. In Gaucher's disease, glucocerebroside increases, due to lack of glucocerebrosidase and in Niemann-Pick disease sphingomyelin is present in excess and in Tay-Sachs disease, ganglioside is the uncatabolised constituent.

A third group of storage diseases is due to failure to remove mucopolysaccaride, the best known being Hurler's syndrome (gargoylism). In this condition chondroitin sulphate and heparitin sulphate accumulate in connective tissue and epithelial cells due to lack of the lysosomal enzyme which normally catabolises them.

Metals may also accumulate to produce a form of storage disease. In hepato-lenticular degeneration, (Wilson's disease) copper accumulates in brain, liver and kidney due to genetically determined lack of a protein that normally binds the metal. In haemochromatosis, the iron pigment haemosiderin is deposited in large amounts in liver, pancreas, skin and other sites. This may be due to a genetically determined lack of iron binding protein and to excessive absorption of iron, genetic or acquired. Haemosiderin may also accumulate due to excessive breakdown of red cells as seen in certain types of anaemia, or after repeated blood transfusion. Haemochromatosis and Wilson's disease may be associated with indolent chronic inflammation, especially in the liver. It seems that the accumulation of heavy metals leads to a slow but steady accumulation of macrophages and to proliferation of fibroblasts and increased synthesis by them of collagen and proteoglycans. A similar situation exists in pneumoconiosis in which silicates in the lung excite a crippling fibrous tissue reaction. Phagocytosis by macrophages is an effective method of neutralising harmful minerals such as copper or silica. Unfortunately the laden phagocytes are provoked to release a variety of active substances one of which is a potent promoter of fibrosis.

Bibliography

Casarett L J, Doull J (ed) 1975 Toxicology: the basic science of poisons. MacMillan, New York

Farber F, Magee P N (eds) 1966 Biochemical pathology. Williams & Wilkins, Baltimore

Keppler D (ed) 1975 Pathogenesis and mechanisms of liver cell necrosis. Medical and Technical Publishing Co, Lancaster

Scarpelli D G, Trump B F 1971 Cell injury. Upjohn Co, Kalamazoo

Tanikawa K 1979 Liver pathology. In: Trump B F, Jones R T (eds) Diagnostic electron microscopy vol 2. Wiley, New York, p 15

23

Dysfunction of the cells of the blood

Erythrocytes

The erythrocytes or red blood corpuscles are by far the most numerous of the cells of the blood. Each mm^3 (microlitre) of blood should contain about 4.5 to 6.2 million red cells. Their importance is that they contain the body's supply of haemoglobin which is required for the transport of oxygen to the tissues, the red cell haemoglobin having become oxygenated in the lungs (p. 172). The important pathology of red cells is the possibility of anaemia, i.e. a deficiency of red cells or haemoglobin in the blood.

There are several different varieties of anaemia each of which in turn depends on a disturbance of some facet of red cell production or metabolism. In addition, each of the main sub-groups usually needs to be further divided to make a comprehensive classification. As in the case of malignant disease (p. 230), the taxonomy of anaemia is not an exercise in memory but an essential prelude to understanding.

Haemolytic anaemias

In this group, anaemia occurs because there is an excessive destruction of red cells. The normal life span of the red corpuscle is about 120 days and the cells when old and effete are destroyed (haemolysed) in the circulation and spleen and liver. It is this process which is exaggerated and accelerated in haemolytic anaemia.

Haemolytic anaemia due to abnormalities of the red cell. The most important numerical group in this category is the diseases due to abnormalities of haemoglobin. This substance which carries the blood oxygen, consists of four haem molecules each bound to a globin polypeptide chain. Most abnormalities of haemoglobin are due to the globin moeity. In sickle cell anaemia (p. 201) the patients, usually of African origin inherit a structural abnormality of the beta chain of the globin in which a glutamic acid molecule is replaced by a valine. This alters the physicochemical nature of the haemoglobin and reduces its solubility. As a result the red cells assume a sickle shape, are rendered fragile and rapidly destroyed in the circulation.

In thalassaemia, an inherited disease of Mediterranean peoples, there is defective synthesis either of beta chains or, less commonly, alpha chains of haemoglobin. The defective chains are replaced by other chains of different structure but once again the red cells are abnormally fragile and rapidly destroyed, leading to anaemia.

Another group of corpuscular defects are due to genetically determined deficiency of intracellular glucose-6-phosphate dehydrogenase (G6PD). This results in impaired activity of the hexosemonophosphate shunt pathway. This leads in turn to failure to generate sufficient energy to maintain glutathione in a reduced state (GSH). GSH itself is needed to maintain the many SH groups of the red cell in a reduced state. Failure to do so makes the cell abnormally permeable. In these groups of disorders, haemolytic anaemia does not usually occur unless precipitated by exposure to an oxidising agent in a drug or foodstuff, e.g. primaquine, sulphonamides, aspirin or the fava bean. The genetics of these disorders are complex, some being sex-linked and occurring in both Mediterranean and African peoples.

The final group of corpuscular haemolytic anaemias arise from abnormal permeability of the red cell membrane. In this category comes hereditary spherocytosis where the cells cannot resist the entry of water and sodium chloride thus becoming spherical and fragile. In this disease, removal of the spleen is often curative because the abnormal corpuscles are no longer destroyed there.

Haemolytic anaemia due to extracorpuscular factors. The most important of these are antibodies. Extrinsic antibodies (alloantibodies) or autologous antibodies (auto-antibodies) can be responsible. In either instance the antibody has the capacity to agglutinate the red cells *in vitro* either directly or after the addition of anti-human globulin (the Coomb's test). In the latter instance the haemolytic antibodies are said to be incomplete. The lack of 'completeness' is however merely a useful laboratory artifact. In the body, the cells are coated with the 'incomplete' IgG which is sufficient to render them highly sensitive to destruction in the spleen and liver and hence to produce a haemolytic anaemia.

The most important haemolytic anaemia due to extrinsic antibodies is that which occurs in a new-born baby which has Rh positive red cells, its mother being Rh negative and having therefore been able to produce antibody to the baby's red cells during fetal life especially during parturition. The antibody-coated red cells of the baby are rapidly haemolysed in the liver and spleen, bile pigment from the broken down haemoglobin stains and damages the basal ganglia of the brain (kernicterus) and death or a spastic child may ensue. It is, however, possible to prevent this catastrophe by injecting a blocking anti-Rh antibody into the mother in the 2 days before delivery.

Haemolytic anaemia may sometimes follow drug sensitisation. Thus penicillin may sometimes act as a haptene (p. 27) with red cell protein and lead to antibody and complement binding and resultant haemolysis.

Auto-immune haemolytic anaemia is by no means rare but in almost no case is its causation clear. It can occur without apparent cause (idiopathic) or as a feature of a wide range of diseases including malignancy such as Hodgkin's disease, other lymphomas or carcinoma or known auto-immune conditions such as systemic lupus erythematosus (p. 54). In most cases the antibodies are of the 'incomplete' variety and haemolysis is due to excessive destruction of the antibody-coated cells by the mononuclear phagocyte system.

Finally, haemolytic auto-antibodies exist which can be demonstrated *in vitro* only by an agglutination reaction performed in the cold, at about O° to 2°C (cold agglutinins). They occur in various diseases, notably mycoplasma pneumonia (p. 6). They are often 'complete' antibodies (see above) and are usually IgM. Unlike all the other antibodies discussed in this section, cold agglutinins usually haemolyse red cells in the circulation by the action of bound activated complement instead of merely rendering them more susceptible to destruction in the spleen and liver.

Iron deficiency anaemia

A major constituent of the haem portion of the haemoglobin molecule is iron. It is obvious therefore that a bodily shortage of iron will lead to an overall deficiency of haemoglobin, i.e. an iron deficiency anaemia. It is equally obvious that iron deficiency might result either from inadequate dietary intake, from inadequate absorption from the intestine or from excessive chronic loss of blood.

When red cells are destroyed at the end of their life span, their organic constituents are broken down, metabolised and excreted. Their iron however is recycled, being taken up by the iron-binding protein apoferritin to form ferritin. As a result, the dietary requirement for iron is low and man has evolved an elaborate mechanism for limiting absorption of inorganic iron. This mechanism consists of the presence in the intestinal epithelium of the protein ferritin which binds ionic iron from the diet and retains it in the intestinal wall.

In situations of chronic blood loss, such as a bleeding peptic ulcer or excessive menstrual bleeding, it has to be assumed either that the diet does not contain sufficient iron to replace that which is being lost, or that the ferritin mechanism is too insensitive to the body's needs to release the iron that is needed. The loss of blood is sometimes massive and prolonged and in such cases iron deficiency anaemia is easily explicable and often readily remedied by dosage with ferrous salts. In other cases the blood loss is modest and the anaemia less explicable. There is certainly evidence that the ferritin mechanism for preventing iron overloading of the body can sometimes be too efficient, in that even when iron deficiency anaemia is present, dietary iron supplements are not absorbed. The diet itself may provide another clue. Poor diets may not contain enough ionic iron, due for example to lack of fresh vegetables. There is, however, another pathway for iron absorption in which the metal is taken up by the intestinal epithelium as part of a relatively intact haem molecule, mainly from the myoglobin of animal protein. From the point of view of iron intake the worst diet would be one lacking both ionic iron and animal protein, the next worse, one lacking only the protein and the best a diet rich in both fresh vegetables and meat. This would be particularly true if, as seems likely, iron absorbed as part of a haem molecule most readily by-passes the excessive restriction imposed on iron absorption when the element is in the ionic form.

Iron deficiency anaemia is a common feature of intestinal malabsorption, e.g. following major by-pass surgery in the intestinal tract. It is often attributed on little evidence, to unavailability of hydrochloric acid, which is thought to promote iron absorption. It is attributed also to excessive speed in the passage of intestinal contents. Its causation is probably more complex than this. It could for example be a consequence of faulty absorption of myoglobin-containing protein, or result from a disturbance of the ferritin iron uptake and discharge mechanism.

Megaloblastic or macrocytic anaemias

Iron can be regarded as an essential nutrient for the production of haemoglobin. The carriage of haemoglobin, however, requires healthy red cells. The formation of healthy corpuscles depends on the usual supply of amino acids, etc. and in theory any severe lack of nutrition should cause red cell production to fail. In practice, iron deficiency supervenes before lack of other dietary constituents becomes effective.

On the other hand, two substances exist which are specifically required for the production of normal red cells, folic acid (pteroylglutamic acid) and vitamin B12 (cyanocobalmin). They are required for the synthesis of nucleic acids, working independently. As might be expected their lack is felt not only by the red cells but also by leucocytes, platelets and indeed may be observed even in epithelial cells. Nevertheless it is the nucleated red cell precursors in the bone marrow which suffer most. When either or both the substances are deficient these cells acquire abnormal nuclei and are called megaloblasts. They give rise to red corpuscles which are larger than normal (macrocytes) but greatly reduced in number so that although each cell carries more than its full complement of haemoglobin the patient is nevertheless severely anaemic. The anaemia is worsened by the undue fragility of the megaloblastic corpuscles which gives rise to an assocaited haemolytic anaemia (p. 162).

The most important cause of megaloblastic anaemia is pernicious anaemia (p. 159) in which atrophy of the mucosa of the upper two-thirds of the stomach leads to absence of a substance called intrinsic factor, essential for the absorption of vitamin B12. Malabsorption from the small intestine is also a common cause of megaloblastic anaemia, often complicated by an associated iron deficiency.

Both folic acid and B12 may be deficient in such states. Such malabsorption may be due to a defect in the intestinal mucosa as in gluten enteropathy (coeliac disease) or to mucosal destruction and inflammation as in Crohn's disease or to growth of abnormal bacterial flora which compete for the dietary folic acid or B12, as may occur after major intestinal surgery.

Aplastic anaemia

In this condition, anaemia develops because the red cell precursors in the bone marrow are absent, destroyed or fail to mature into red corpuscles, even of the abnormal variety. It is essentially depression or destruction of the haemopoetic tissue in the bone marrow and as might be expected is likely to affect not only red cells, but also leucocytes and platelets, causing a so-called pancytopaenia.

The commonest cause is toxic depression of the marrow as occurs for example in chronic renal failure (uraemia, azotaemia) where retained metabolites prevent normal marrow function. Lack of erythropoetin, the red-cell stimulating factor formed in the kidney (p. 93) has been invoked as a cause and may play a contributory but minor role.

Many drugs have the unfortunate side effect of causing aplastic anaemia, e.g. benzene or cytotoxic drugs used in cancer chemotherapy. Other common drugs cause the disease in only a few susceptible individuals. In this category come chloramphenicol, gold salts and phenylbutazone. Ionising radiation is of course an important cause of marrow aplasia (p. 183). Sometimes, the bone marrow becomes so heavily infiltrated by malignant cells, that the erythropoetic cells are destroyed and replaced and aplastic anaemia results. A similar result may follow fibrosis or bony replacement of the marrow spaces due to diseases of obscure nature, e.g. myelofibrosis.

Leucocytes

These are the 'white' (i.e. non-haemoglobin containing) cells of the circulation. They consist of the polymorphonuclear leucocytes or granulocytes (comprising neutrophils, eosinophils and basophils according to their staining characteristics and in descending order of importance), the lymphocytes and the monocytes. All types of leucocytes can rise or fall in number in the circulation as a result of disease. With the exception of malignant transformation (leukaemia), a rise in number is called a leucocytosis, monocytosis or lymphocytosis and a fall in number a leucopenia, etc.

Polymorphonuclear leucocytes

These are the highly important phagocytes discussed elsewhere (p. 17). The subject of polymorph leucocytosis also is dealt with elsewhere (p. 95). Lymphocytosis is a less important phenomenon seen mainly in viral diseases such as infectious mononucleosis. Monocytosis is unimportant.

Leucopenia

Leucocytes, unlike red corpuscles do not appear to fall in number because of excessive destruction or, with the exception of B12 and folate deficiency, because of nutritional factors. A leucopenia is almost always the result of toxic depression of polymorph precursors in the bone marrow. The causes of such a depression are the same as those already listed for precipitating aplastic anaemia. By far the most important is the use of the cytotoxic antimetabolites, such as cyclophosphamide or methotrexate, used in the chemotherapy of cancer, but there are also rare leucopenias of unknown aetiology. There are normally about 4000 neutrophil polymorphs per microlitre (mm^3) of blood. This level needs to fall to about 400 to make serious infection a likely consequence and to about 200 before acute inflammatory reactions containing substantial numbers of the cells cease to be produced. Lymphopenia and monocytopenia are unimportant except as complications of malignant disease.

Leukaemia

This is a neoplastic proliferation of leucocytes and their precursors in the bone marrow and can be regarded as the result of malignant transformation (p. 250) of these cells. It may affect the polymorphonuclear (myeloid), lymphocytic or monocytic populations, the last being relatively uncommon.

Leukaemia exists in two forms, acute (blastic) or chronic (cytic). Thus it is customary to refer to myeloblastic, myelocytic, lymphoblastic, lymphocytic leukaemia. The essential difference between acute and chronic leukaemias is the presence in the circulation in the acute variety of very primitive leucocyte precursors, i.e. myeloblasts or lymphoblasts. As might be expected from the terminology, in the absence of treatment acute leukaemia would normally lead to death more rapidly than the chronic variety. However, with treatment many cases of 'acute' lymphatic leukaemia now have a better prospect of survival than many cases of 'chronic' myeloid leukaemia.

The uncontrolled proliferation of leukaemic cells in the bone marrow often spills over to the circulation and causes very high leucocyte counts, sometimes exceeding 100 000 per microlitre (mm^3) of blood. There are often deposits of the neoplastic leucocytes in many organs and tissues. More importantly, the replacement of normal bone marrow leads to severe anaemia and deficiency of circulating platelets (see below). In addition, a mysterious haemolytic anaemia due to autoantibodies (p. 54) may complicate the clinical situation. Paradoxically, all leukaemic patients are very susceptible to infection because of lack of bactericidal capability (p. 24). In blastic leukaemias there may indeed be very few mature granulocytes in the circulation but in chronic myeloid leukaemia it has to be presumed that the enormous numbers of polymorphs in the blood do not possess the antimicrobial activity of their normal counterparts.

Leukaemia is known to be provoked by exposure to ionising radiation and in birds and rodents and other mammals to be due to oncogenic viruses (p. 246). The search for a viral aetiology in man has not yet borne fruit. Many cases of chronic myeloid leukamia exhibit an abnormal chromosome number 22 (the Philadelphia chromosome) in their marrow cells and in Down's syndrome (trisomy 21) there is a greatly increased incidence of acute myeloid leukaemia. The nature of these links with specific chromosome abnormalities remains obscure.

Platelets
These cells play a major role in thrombosis and have been discussed elsewhere (p. 140) in that capacity. Their numbers in the circulation, apart from some cases of rare diseases such as polycythaemia rubra vera increase only as a transient phenomenon, e.g. after injury.

There are, however, many pathological situations in which the number of circulating platelets falls. This is serious, because the cells are vital for the prevention of bleeding from capillaries. It seems likely that they are required continuously to form haemostatic plugs in these tiny vessels. When their numbers fall below about 60 000 per microlitre of blood (the normal number being 120 000 to 600 000) spontaneous haemorrhages (purpura) take place in brain, skin, mucous

membranes, intestinal tract, lungs and elsewhere and fatal haemorrhage is likely to occur.

The commonest cause of platelet deficiency (thrombocytopenia) is
damage to the multinucleate platelet precursor in the bone marrow,
the megakaryocyte, by anti-metabolic drugs used in cancer chemotherapy. Similar bone marrow effects are produced by the physical and
chemical agents which cause aplastic anaemia, for example ionising
radiation or benzene poisoning. Thrombocytopenia is also a major
feature of leukaemia, due mostly to replacement of megakaryocytes by
neoplastic cells.

In addition to the destruction or replacement of megokaryocytes,
thrombocytopenia is a well recognised consequence of hypersensitivity to certain drugs, notably sedormid or quinidine. The drug acts as a
haptene in combining with platelets and the cells are destroyed by
complement activated by the adherent antibody provoked by the
drug/platelet combination. This is a classical example of type II
hypersensitivity (p. 44).

Needless to say there are several diseases in which circulating
platelets are few in number for no known cause. The most important of
these is idiopathic thrombocytopenic purpura, which is often
relieved by removal of the spleen. Another important cause of purpura
of obscure pathogenesis is chronic renal failure (uraemia or azotaemia). The platelets are of normal numbers but there is evidence of
abnormal function i.e. small wounds take an unduly long time to stop
bleeding (prolonged bleeding time). It seems likely that retained toxic
metabolites interfere with platelet function in some way and massive
spontaneous haemorrhage, often from the bowel, is a common terminal
event in those dying of kidney failure.

Bibliography

Thompson R B 1979 A short textbook of haematology 5th edn. Pitman, Tunbridge
  Wells

24

Failure of body systems

Heart failure

Cardiac failure occurs when the heart is unable to pump blood at a rate adequate for the needs of the tissues. It is also known as congestive cardiac failure, chronic congestive cardiac failure or passive venous congestion. These terms draw attention to the accumulation of blood in the venous system which is a feature of inadequate cardiac output. Cardiac failure implies a primary derangement of the heart. Inadequate cardiac output due to diminished venous return as a result of fall in blood volume (hypovolaemia) is a feature of shock and is dealt with elsewhere (p. 113).

Cardiac failure occurs because there is either a primary failure of heart muscle, e.g. after a cardiac infarct or because an intolerable burden is thrown upon the muscle, e.g. by high blood pressure or disease of the heart valves. The initial response to an increased burden is increased output achieved by dilatation of the ventricles and enlargement of their muscle fibres so that the capacity and force of the pump are increased (p. 191). Eventually, however, the adaptive process ceases to be effective and output falls. The reasons for this are uncertain. One explanation is that the enlarged muscle fibres need more blood from the coronary arteries to keep them functioning and if this blood flow proves inadequate the muscle will fail. In practice, one ventricle usually fails before the other, depending on the cause. Primary lung disease which increases the resistance to the outflow from the right ventricle initiates right ventricular failure. Practically all other heart disease initiates left-sided failure. In left-sided failure, venous blood accumulates first in the pulmonary circulation which drains into the left atrium. Falling left ventricular output causes diminished glomerular blood flow which is wrongly interpreted by the kidney as reduced blood volume so that sodium and chloride are reabsorbed to excess, partly because of increased secretion of aldosterone by the adrenal cortex. As a result of this retention of salt, water is trapped in the tissues thus adding to the problems of the failing heart. Retention of salt and water in response to a temporary fall in blood volume due to blood loss would be a survival mechanism for a hunting mammal and has probably evolved as such. The same mechanism, however, acts very much to the disadvantage of the middle aged or elderly patient with cardiac disease.

Failure of the right ventricle leads to venous congestion in the systemic circulation, which normally drains into the right atrium. This affects especially the subcutaneous tissues, liver, spleen and kidneys. Venous congestion of the kidney again causes diminished glomerular filtration of blood with the consequences given above. Passive congestion of the systemic circulation, due to right ventricular failure throws a severe load on the left ventricle and congestion of the lungs, due to left ventricular failure burdens the right ventricle. Commonly therefore both sides of the heart become involved sooner or later in the process of cardiac failure. In addition, the combination of lessened arterial perfusion with venous engorgement interferes with the function of many other organs, notably the lungs and kidney but also the brain and liver, and a multiple self-reinforcing systems failure may occur as a prelude to death.

Liver failure

General failure of liver function is less predictable in nature than cardiac failure. Jaundice, due to accumulation in the blood of bilirubin which the damaged liver cells cannot excrete, is a fairly constant manifestation although there are many other causes of jaundice. Inability to synthesise albumin and other plasma proteins is also seen and in the later stages failure of prothrombin synthesis develops, with resultant bleeding. Leakage of mitochondrial enzymes into the circulation occurs and there is progressive failure to conjugate and hydroxylate drugs and metabolites so that toxic effects develop, especially in the brain, the patients often dying in coma.

Failure of intestinal function

Apart from blockage or inadequate peristalsis, the most important manifestation of cellular dysfunction in the intestine is inability to digest and absorb food. This leads to a malabsorption syndrome which may take a variety of forms but usually results in anaemia, deficiencies of vitamins, and disturbances of protein, fat and carbohydrate metabolism.

Renal failure

The kidney's role in homeostasis is so vital that any disturbance in its function is soon relected in the body fluids and any major impairment is incompatible with life. Acute renal failure is usually associated with a failure to form urine and most commonly follows severe impairment of renal blood flow. Metabolites accumulate, electrolyte and acid base equilibrium cannot be maintained and the patient dies if no relief is forthcoming.

Chronic renal failure usually occurs as a result of long lasting kidney disease and commonly involves both glomerular filtration and tubular function. Failure to reabsorb water may be an early feature and this is likely to be complicated by retention of sodium. Acidosis, associated with an inability to form ammonium ions is commonly seen and also depletion of blood calcium. Nitrogenous waste products, notably urea, accumulate in the blood and a variety of toxic effects result in which the lungs, brain, heart, bone marrow and gastrointestinal tract may suffer. Death is inevitable unless an artificial system for maintaining homeostasis is used (renal dialysis) or a renal transplant performed.

Respiratory failure

In biology, respiration is the process whereby cells obtain energy by the processes of oxidation or glycolysis. Oxidative respiration involves the transport of oxygen and carbon dioxide to and from the cell via the circulation and their entry and discharge via specialised organs. In man and other mammals this latter process entails the entry of atmospheric air into the alveolar spaces of the lung and *vice versa* and the exchange of oxygen and carbon dioxide between the alveolar air and the blood in the alveolar capillaries. In pathology, the term respiratory failure refers normally to those processes which occur in the lung. Since this is mainly gaseous exchange, respiratory failure is commonly defined as an abnormally low oxygen tension in arterial blood, the critical value being a Po_2 of less than 60 mm Hg or a rise in arterial carbon dioxide to a Pco_2 of 50 mm Hg or more.

There are two main causes of respiratory insufficiency, inadequate ventilation of the lungs and inadequate gas exchange at the blood air barrier (the alveolar wall). In underventilation, the main effect is a raised arterial Pco_2 and a resultant acidosis. The arterial Po_2 falls but not usually to a sufficient degree to cause serious difficulty. Inadequate ventilation occurs in obstructive airways disease, i.e. chronic bronchitis or asthma and also as a result of interference with movement of the respiratory muscles, e.g. in partial paralysis. Total paralysis leads of course to death.

In impaired gas exchange there is a reduction in the surface available for the passage of oxygen and carbon dioxide, i.e. at the alveolar wall. This occurs commonly in emphysema and severe chronic bronchitis and in a wide variety of diseases where lung tissue is destroyed and replaced by fibrous tissue. A common underlying cause of inadequate gas exchange is an imbalance between perfusion and ventilation. In other words those parts of the lung which receive an adequate supply of blood may not be adequately ventilated by air. This happens when there is a severe disturbance of lung architecture, due to destructive disease processes such as emphysema (overdistension and damage to alveoli).

The most important effect of this type of respiratory failure is interference with oxygen uptake, a fall in arterial Po_2 and the appearance of cyanosis, i.e. blueness of the skin and mucous membranes due to excessive amounts of reduced haemoglobin in the capillaries. By contrast, carbon dioxide elimination is much less impaired. In practice, it is common to see both types of respiratory failure coexisting since chronic bronchitis often goes hand in hand with emphysema.

Respiratory failure may lead to right-sided heart failure because of increased resistance to blood flow through the lungs. This may be due to vascular obliteration after pulmonary destruction and fibrosis, pulmonary vasoconstriction (secondary to abnormalities in alveolar gaseous tension) or abnormal arterio-venous shunts. At first the right ventricle hypertrophies as a compensatory mechanism (p. 191) but then eventually dilates and fails (cor pulmonale).

Bibliography

Sodeman W A Jr, Sodeman W A (eds) 1979 Pathologic physiology 6th edn. Saunders, Philadelphia

25

Oedema

Oedema is the abnormal accumulation of fluid in the extravascular and extracellular compartments of the body. Fluid normally enters this compartment from the small blood vessels, mainly venules and capillaries although arterioles may also participate, at least in the lung. Its entry is controlled locally by a number of opposing forces, in particular the balance between hydrostatic and oncotic pressures (Starling's hypothesis).

Three factors are important; the height of the hydrostatic pressure in the capillaries, which tends to increase filtration; the oncotic pressure of the plasma proteins which retain water and inhibit filtration; the state of permeability of the vessel wall. Other factors of less importance are the tissue tension of the extravascular space which limits filtration if high, and the efficiency of lymphatic drainage which removes fluid from the extravascular compartment.

There are many situations in pathology in which oedema occurs and in most of these the mechanisms are complex and often not fully understood. Nevertheless, there are in essence only three types of oedema; the inflammatory, the hydrostatic and the lymphatic.

Inflammatory oedema

This has been dealt with elsewhere (p. 60). It is due to altered permeability of the venular and capillary wall so that protein which is normally retained in the circulation is allowed to escape into the tissues. Once there, it retains water with it and will remain until the vessels cease to leak protein and the exudate can be removed by lymphatic drainage. It is important to appreciate that once vessel walls leak protein, Starling's laws can no longer apply, because they assume a vessel almost impermeable to plasma protein. Nevertheless the loss of protein-rich fluid (fluid exudate) is doubtless accelerated by the rise in hydrostatic pressure which may be present in the inflamed vessels. Similarly, oedema will be restricted if the local tissue tension is high, as it is for example in the palms of the hands, or facilitated if tension is low, as in the loose subcutaneous tissue of the ankle. The commonest cause of inflammatory oedema is bacterial infection, but other common causes are hypersensitivity (p. 43) or irritation by chemicals, heat, trauma or (in the lungs) gases. Rarely, the mediators which increase vascular permeability become activated and cause oedema as a result of hereditary deficiencies of enzymes or inhibitors (familial angio-oedema).

Hydrostatic oedema

By contrast, this occurs as a result of disturbances in the balancing forces governing fluid transport when vascular permeability is normal. It is an important feature of cardiac and renal failure (p. 170). It is usually complex in its pathogenesis. Generalised oedema is prominent in right-sided heart failure. As the right ventricle fails in its pumping action, the pressure in the systemic veins which drain into the right atrium rises. As a result there is increased filtration of fluid especially into lax tissues like the ankle or sacrum or into tissue spaces such as the pleural space. Normally however this increase could be dealt with by lymphatic drainage and excreted via the kidney. Unfortunately, the underperfusion of the kidney which occurs in heart failure leads to retention of sodium partly as a direct consequence of lowered glomerular filtration, partly because of inappropriate aldosterone production. Retention of sodium inevitably entails retention of water, so oedema persists. The importance of the kidney in this situation is readily demonstrated by the rapid disappearance of oedema which occurs in such patients after administration of drugs whose only action is to increase excretion of water and sodium.

In renal disease, oedema is most prominent when the main symptoms consist of massive loss of protein in the urine due to glomerular disease. This loss is followed by a fall in plasma protein concentration especially of albumin (the nephrotic syndrome). Presumably, therefore, some loss of fluid into the tissues occurs because the oncotic pressure of the plasma, which depends mainly on albumin, falls below the level needed to counteract the hydrostatic pressure in the capillaries. However, as in heart failure, the kidney is underperfused, this time because of glomerular disease, so once again sodium is retained, with consequent persistence of oedema. There is also reduction in plasma volume which further stimulates aldosterone release and also that of antidiuretic hormone. Hydrostatic oedema occurs in hepatic cirrhosis and liver failure and in malnutrition and in endocrine disorders. The pathogenesis is invariably complex and usually involves the renal regulation of fluid as well as disturbances in Starling's equation.

A more simple example of hydrostatic oedema may be seen after occlusion of a major leg vein by thrombus (p. 143). Here blockage of the vein leads to a rise in pressure distal to the obstruction with increased filtration pressure. As a result there is some local oedema but its extent and duration are variable.

Lymphatic oedema

Oedema due to lack of lymphatic drainage occurs in a variety of situations. It may contribute to the accumulation of fluid in the peritoneal cavity seen in hepatic cirrhosis. It may occur in the legs as a result of congenital abnormalities in the lymphatic channels (Milroy's disease). It may follow lymphatic blockage by filariae in helminth infections or may develop when lymphatic vessels are obstructed by tumour. In all these situations, entry of fluid into the extravascular space may be normal and only its removal by lymphatic drainage impaired.

Pulmonary oedema

When fluid accumulates in the lungs it does so first in the alveolar walls then in the air spaces, so that ultimately the patient may literally drown. Pulmonary oedema may be due either to inflammatory or hydrostatic mechanisms or to both. The oedema of left-sided heart failure probably results from a shift of blood from the systemic to the pulmonary circulation, rather than simple uncomplicated increase in filtration pressure in the pulmonary veins draining into the left ventricle. This shift seems to be a particular consequence of systemic hypertension and is aggravated by any sympathomimetic stimulus, e.g. anxiety. It can be simulated experimentally by giving adrenalin or by damage to the nervous system. It is probably for these reasons that pulmonary oedema may occur after head injuries or cranial operations. A similar shift of blood from the systemic to the pulmonary circuit may explain the oedema of the lungs which often develops as a terminal event in many diseases, e.g. renal failure. Inflammatory pulmonary oedema occurs in bacterial or viral infections of the lung or after exposure to noxious gases. The pulmonary oedema which occurs after severe trauma (shock lung) probably results from a combination of hydrostatic and inflammatory effects.

Bibliography

Hurley J V 1978 Current views on the mechanisms of pulmonary oedema. Journal of Pathology 125: 59

Intaglietta M, Johnson P C 1978 Principles of capillary exchange. In: Johnson P C (ed) Peripheral circulation. Wiley, New York, P 141

26

Nutritional pathology

Pressure on the world's food resources, an awareness by the well fed of the prevalence of malnutrition in their own and in other countries, and general anxiety about what foods are or are not necessary make the pathology of nutrition a topical subject.

For adequate nutrition, two criteria must be fulfilled; sufficient daily inatke of calories and a satisfactory consumption of certain essential dietary ingredients. The calorie needs of an average adult are about 2500 per 24 hours, but may be much more or much less depending on who he is, where he lives, what he does and how old he is. Children and young people have higher requirements of almost everything including calories. If young people do not receive adequate food they will in later life be at a permanent disadvantage with their contemporaries who were fed properly when young. This is because the developing brain in particular has higher nutritional needs. The importance of nutrition in early life should make us sceptical of attributing differences in intelligence between races or socio-economomic groups to inherited superiority or inferiority.

The simplest type of malnutrition and the easiest to correct is a shortage of calories with no major imbalance in the dietary constituents. In children this produces a picture of generalised wasting known as marasmus, which is a medical euphemism for starvation. A young infant needs about 100 calories per kg of body weight per day and the figure declines slowly to the adult level of about 30 calories.

A more complicated situation occurs when total calorie intake is sufficient but the diet is deficient in other respects. There are about 50 organic and inorganic substances which the body cannot synthesise for itself but must receive in the diet ready made and in adequate amounts. These ingredients are distributed over the four main groups of food, i.e. meat, milk, cereal and vegetables and the further diet deviates from a balanced mixture of all four, the more difficult does proper nutrition become.

Protein is vital because the body cannot dispense with its need for the eight essential amino acids, lysine, phenylalanine, methionine, leucine, isoleucine, tryptophane, threonine and valine. A protein with all these amino acids in proper amounts has a biological value of 100 per cent. A protein with a biological value of 60 per cent or less can never fulfil the body's needs for amino acids no matter how much is eaten. This is why man cannot live on bread alone although the cereal from which it is made contains much protein. Similar cereals fed to cattle, however, are converted to meat which has a biological value of 100 per cent.

Plans to wean man away from his expensive habit of eating meat depend therefore on providing an alternative source of protein with a biological value approximating to 100 per cent. Since man needs about 0.5 to 1.0 g of protein per kg body weight every day, i.e. must have about 5 per cent of his total calories in the form of high grade protein, this is not an easy task. In primitive societies men may solve the problem partially by eating large amounts of two or more proteins of lower biological value which with luck will complement their respective amino acid deficiencies. This is a very inefficient solution and one may wonder whether man would have achieved his spectacular evolutionary success if he had not become carnivorous. Gorillas need to spend most of their waking hours eating, in order to take in adequate amounts of essential dietary ingredients. This must make them very vulnerable in terms of natural selection.

Unfortunately, large sections of the world's population are obliged by necessity to resort to a similar expedient, but with limited success. The outcome of a diet adequate in total calories but lacking in high-quality protein is a disease called kwashiorkor, from a Ghanaian word meaning 'second child', i.e. those deprived of breast feeding at too early an age. Children with kwashiorkor are stunted and pot-bellied and show the predictable consequences of having insufficient amino acids with which to build protein, e.g. anaemia, low plasma albumin, abnormalities of skin and hair and a fatty liver (because they cannot synthesise lipoprotein p. 158). Kwashiorkor is rarely a pure protein deficiency and if this is corrected by giving skimmed milk, more harm than good may follow, because other deficiencies especially in vitamins, may be unmasked, particularly if the requirement for them is increased by a protein-induced spurt of growth.

Protein lack is often accompanied by deficiencies in the vitamin B complex, including thiamine, riboflavine and niacin. These vitamins are needed only in very small amounts but are vital for the processes of cellular respiration which generate the energy on which life depends. Lack of thiamine in the diet causes the disease of beri-beri, due partly to direct lack of thiamine and partly to accumulation of toxic amounts of pyruvate as a result of thiamine deficiency. In beri-beri the heart, skeletal muscle, brain and nerves are affected, since these have the highest energy needs. Niacin (nicotinamide), like thiamine is an essential constituent of some of the molecules which carry out cell respiration. Its absence from the diet leads to the disease of pellagra, associated with dementia, diarrhoea and dermatitis. Riboflavin deficiency is again usually part of a general malnutrition and leads to abnormalities in the skin, tongue and eyes.

Deficiency of vitamin C occurs mainly when the diet is lacking in fresh fruit, vegetables or meat. Ascorbic acid is required for the synthesis of collagen and proteoglycans (p. 81) and most of the effects of vitamin C deficiency (scurvy) can be attributed to connective tissue defects. These result in haemorrhage from fragile blood vessels, defective growth of bone and teeth and poor healing of wounds. In view of recent publicity, it is interesting that the volunteer who in 1940 put himself on a diet totally lacking in vitamin C in order to determine the time needed for scurvy to develop, reported a remarkable absence of head colds during the 3 winter months before his scorbutic symptoms began.

Lack of vitamin D is a consequence of malnutrition in countries not noted for sunshine, since in sunny countries the vitamin is synthesised in the skin by the action of ultra violet light. Vitamin D is present in many foods and lack of it produces rickets, a disease of bone growth common in industrialised societies before the days of prosperity and the welfare state. Rickets is due to a failure to deposit minerals in bone, so that they become softened and the role of vitamin D is probably to regulate the metabolism of calcium and phosphate and thus to enable the mineralisation to occur. As might be expected therefore, lack of calcium and phosphate in the diet also causes rickets.

Inadequate intake of the other fat soluble vitamins A, E and K are more likely to be seen in intestinal disease than as a result of dietary deficiencies. The malabsorption syndrome (p. 171) is particularly liable to interfere with the intake of these vitamins, including vitamin D.

The other important dietary constituent which is prone to deficiency is iron. Lack of iron is as common as inadequate protein intake, which is not surprising since meat is the major dietary source of iron. Shortage of meat and the low efficiency of iron absorption from the intestine combine to produce this deficit. Iron deficiency produces anaemia but it is suspected that it has other effects on the body which are not yet clear.

Obesity

There is no difficulty in recognising an obese person, but some problem in defining the term. The best definition is probably a body weight 30 per cent or more above the norm for a particular height. The norms which act as a reference point are usually based on figures derived originally from the Metropolitan Life Insurance Co. of the United States. As examples, in this tabulation, the 'normal' weight of a woman 1.6 m in height is 116 kg and that of a man 1.72 m in height is 145 kg. The excess body weight of the obese person is mainly fat. Heavy-framed people with above average muscular development but no excess of fat cannot properly be called obese and in practice are unlikely to exceed the 'norm' by more than 20 per cent.

Obesity consists largely of an increase in the triglyceride stored in the fat depots of the body, especially in subcutaneous tissue. Attempts to measure obesity by estimating skinfold thickness, e.g. over the triceps muscle of the arm, have however led to conflicting results. The excess fat is deposited as a result of an increase in the size, i.e. hypertrophy (p. 191) of the fat cells or lipocytes. It is only when obesity develops early in life that fat cells also increase in number (hyperplasia).

The relationship of body water to obesity has led to some confusion. When an obese person begins a starvation diet the body fat is broken down eventually to CO_2 and water. Thus one mole of a fatty acid, e.g. palmitic acid yields after oxidation a net 32 g of water. This water is excreted by diuresis so that most of the initial weight loss may appear to be due to loss of water. In some cases the water is retained for a period, so that the initial response of obesity to starvation may be a discouraging but transient weight gain.

Nevertheless, although about 70 per cent of the excess weight in obesity is almost always due to fat, a modest increase in body water, protein and carbohydrate may also occur.

The pathogenesis of obesity is always the same, i.e. an excess of calorie intake over calorie expenditure. In other words, obese subjects obey the law of conservation of energy. Energy expenditure can be measured by estimating O_2 consumption and CO_2 output with a correction for urinary nitrogen (derived from utilised protein). Calorie intake is of course easily measured. It can be shown by studying these equations that however little obese patients eat, their energy expenditure is even less.

The tendency of people to increase in weight with the onset of middle age is due partly to diminished bodily activity. In addition, however, the calories required to maintain a given body weight diminish by about 5 per cent for every decade of life, due presumably to changing patterns of growth, endocrine function and ageing. Factors which increase the number of calories required to maintain a constant weight are thyroid hormone, pituitary growth hormone, androgens, adrenalin and noradrenalin. Thus an excess of any of these factors will lead to loss of weight or to increased intake of food.

Since it is due to an excess of intake over expenditure, it is predictable that obesity can be due to defects in the regulation of both calorie utilisation and of food intake. It is possible that hormones could work directly on fat cells to induce hypertrophy and this may account for certain characteristic patterns of obesity, e.g. in Cushing's syndrome. In general, however, even where a specific hormone can be implicated as in myxoedema (thyroid deficiency), there is demonstrable diminution in energy expenditure. In most cases of obesity associated with low calorie utilisation no specific hormone defect can be found. However, strains of obese mice exist in which low energy expenditure is inherited in Mendelian fashion and much human obesity may be due to a similar mechanism. The suggestion that people are obese because their fat deposits are defective in releasing or metabolising fatty acids now seems to be unsubstantiated except in a few rare cases. On the other hand, there is now some evidence that a relatively high proportion of brown fat, which releases its stored calories more readily than white fat, is a protective factor against obesity.

Energy utilisation is one side of the equation, but calorie intake is the other. Although there is individual variation in calorie needs, this should be balanced by corresponding differences in food intake. People may have normal, subnormal or (less likely) supernormal energy utilisation and be obese because of a food intake which is even slightly excessive for their needs.

Food intake is regulated by two centres in the hypothalamus. These are probably an alpha adrenergic feeding centre which increases appetite and a beta adrenergic 'satiety' centre which switches it off. Normally these centres recognise the metabolic needs of the individual by mechanisms as yet obscure and regulate appetite and food intake accordingly. In many obese patients, however, food intake is regulated not so much by metabolic need as by psychological stimuli such as oral gratification and the taste, availability and appearance of food.

It is well recognised by insurance companies that obesity shortens expectation of life. Obesity leads to hyperinsulinaemia and such patients require more insulin than normal subjects to utilise a given amount of glucose. Obesity is therefore a cause of Type II diabetes mellitus (p. 226). It is also closely linked with hypertension, ischaemic heart disease and atheroma. These links are complex since obesity may be associated with diminished activity and excessive food intake, an unduly high proportion of which is likely to be lipid. All these are risk factors for ischaemic heart disease (p. 135).

If there is a genetic basis for some obesity it is surprising for the trait to have survived so long since obese subjects probably have a slightly lower reproductive rate than their slimmer counterparts. In fact, assuming a normal food intake, obesity represents the state of highest efficiency for calorie utilisation, in that a high proportion of the energy intake is stored. Moreover the energy is stored in fat cells which yield 7 calories/g wet weight as opposed to 1.5 calories/g wet weight of muscle cells. When food is scarce it is not hard to see the survival advantage of the type of obesity associated with normal food intake and low energy utilisation. Certainly there are examples of such individuals surviving starvation conditions, e.g. in wartime, while most others succumbed. This interesting genetic speculation is however of little importance in Western society relative to the increased mortality associated with over-eating and diminished physical activity.

Bibliography

Bray G A 1979 Nutritional factors in disease. In: Soderman and Soderman (eds) Pathological physiology 6th edn. Saunders, Philadelphia, p 971

Davidson S, Passmore R, Brock J F (eds) 1972 Human nutrition and dietetics 5th edn. Churchill Livingstone, Edinburgh

W.H.O. Chronical 1974 28: no. 3

27

Pathology caused by ionising radiation

Ionising radiation (radioactivity) like malnutrition is a topical and important subject. It is a serious form of injury which produces many different effects depending on dosage, duration of exposure, site of damage and type of radiation. X-rays are perhaps the best known form of radioactivity and are generated by machines designed for the purpose. Like gamma rays they are a form of electromagnetic radiation but the latter are emitted spontaneously by the decay of radioactive materials such as radium. Other forms of radioactivity include alpha particles, beta particles (electrons), neutrons and protons. All these are particles of known mass and charge given off by radioactive substances, atomic reactions or particle accelerators.

Radioactivity is widely used in medicine in the form of radiotherapy for cancer. The principle is that the cancer is destroyed by the rays or particles used, while the adjacent normal tissue is preserved. The susceptibility of cancer cells is related to the special ability of radiant energy to damage rapidly dividing cells while having much less effect on other cells. There are, however, many exceptions to this rule in that some rapidly growing cancers are resistant to radiotherapy and some slow growing tumours are remarkably susceptible. In some instances there are explanations other than variation in cellular susceptibility for these discrepancies, e.g. awkward location or low oxygen concentration at the site of the tumour.

If enough radioactivity is deployed every cell type in the body is vulnerable. In practice, however, after acute accidental exposure of the whole body the lymphoid tissue, bone marrow, intestine and gonads are those usually affected, since these are where the most rapidly dividing cells are situated. There is a dramatic fall in the number of circulating lymphocytes, although the levels often return to normal within a few weeks provided the patient survives. The effect on the bone marrow is more serious, for granulocyte production may fall to zero and it may be months later before circulating granulocytes return to normal numbers. Platelet production suffers a similar blow and so does the generation of red blood cells. The results are catastrophic since the patient may bleed to death from lack of platelets (p. 168) and is completely susceptible to infection due to absence of granulocytes (p. 167). In the slightly longer term deprivation of lymphocytes may hamper antibody production and aggravate the risk of infection (p. 41).

The intestine suffers badly from radioactivity since the rapidly dividing intestinal epithelial cells are very vulnerable. It is common for severely irradiated patients to die of intractable diarrhoea. Even carcinoma of the intestine is less sensitive to radiant energy than normal intestinal epithelium, possibly because cell division in the tumour is usually slower than in the normal epithelium, cancerous growth occurring in spite of this paradox .

The gonads contain many rapidly dividing cells and it is therefore not surprising that they may suffer irreparable damage from radiant energy. The ovaries often fare worse than the testes, but patients of both sexes are liable to be made infertile.

Another organ likely to suffer immediately, especially in very severe nuclear energy accidents, is the brain, patients often dying in convulsions. Neurones themselves are fairly radio-resistant as might be predicted from their low capacity for mitosis. The effects of large doses of radiation on the brain are therefore attributable to anoxia due to damage to cerebral blood vessels.

In general, the endothelium of the small blood vessels suffer badly from irradiation injury. The cells swell or disintegrate and this is followed by proliferation of endothelium and fibroblasts with subsequent reduction in blood supply. The lungs may be severely damaged by irradiation, showing exudation of fluid followed by scarring. These effects (radiation pneumonitis) are due at least partly to injury to the small blood vessels of the lung. Post-irradiation changes in the kidney (radiation nephritis) may be the result of a similar train of events.

The cancer-inducting effects of radioactivity are mentioned elsewhere (p. 262) and this represents a serious late sequel to irradiation. It usually occurs in the bone marrow or in organs, e.g. the thyroid, given small doses for some other reason. Twenty years or more may elapse before this effect is seen. Other delayed effects of small doses or of larger doses from which the patient recovered, are cataract of the eye, disappearance of blood cell precursors from the bone marrow (aplastic anaemia), and developmental defects in children who were irradiated while in their mother's uterus.

Clinically, the effects observed in the lungs and kidneys usually occur in the medium term after quite high doses. The effects in the brain are seen usually only after very high doses to the whole body. The effects on the rapidly proliferating cell populations of the bone marrow, lymphoid tissue and gonads and intestines are seen after modest doses applied either locally or to the whole body. If the doses are high, however, the patient may not live long enough to discover that he is sterile.

There is no known safe lower threshold dose for the long term effects of radiation but for acute whole body irradiation, effects on lymphoid tissue, bone marrow and intestines are apparent at 100 rads and at 1000 rads damage to them will cause death within a few weeks. At a dose of 10000 rads to the whole body, death will ensue in a few hours due to brain damage. However, it requires about 1 million rads to kill some bacteria and 10 million rads to ensure death of all living organisms. The rad (R) is a measure of the quantity of radiant energy absorbed by a gram of tissue. As might be expected from its name, ionising radiation damages cells by causing the formation of charged ions from the various molecules which make up the cells structural and functional units. Such ionisation produces changes in the affected molecules which makes it impossible for them to function properly. The nucleus of the cell is the principle target, again predictable from the susceptibility of cell populations in mitosis. The molecular target is DNA which may itself be attacked or which may suffer as a result of a primary attack on messenger RNA leading to a failure of DNA replicating enzymes. Apart from massive doses of about 10000 rads the fundamental effect of ionising radiation on cells is inhibition of DNA synthesis with the inevitable sequel of interference with cell division. Disruption of DNA synthesis may present as disappearance of a cell population (since the cells can no longer replace themselves) degeneration or accelerated death of cells (since they cannot produce essential constituents) or chromosomal abnormalities (structural evidence of damage to DNA molecules). DNA in process of replication is more vulnerable to ionising radiation than resting DNA, again a predictable circumstance from the demonstrable susceptibility of dividing cell populations. The susceptibility of the replicating DNA molecule to radiation may reflect a general inability of DNA which is reproducing itself to withstand even mildly unfavourable circumstances without acquiring chemical faults. The ease with which DNA replication deviates from normal is disadvantageous as regards radiation but is also the basis of mutation, natural selection and evolution (p. 198).

Ionisation of the chemical constituents of cells is achieved by transfer of energy from the ionising radiation so that electrons are displaced from the atoms and molecules of the cell components. This could be a direct effect on DNA or other substances. It is perhaps more important that the ionising radiation leads to the formation of highly reactive free radicles within the cell which in turn cause damage to cell constituents, for example by causing peroxidation. Intracellular water readily yields free radicles such as H^+ or OH^- and for this reason, and because it is the major cell constituent, water may be the main primary target for radioactive emissions.

Bibliography

Coggle J E, Noakes G R 1971 Biological effects of radiation. Wykeham Publication

Pizzarello D J, Witcofski R L 1972 Medical radiation biology Lea & Febinger, Philadelphia

White D C 1975 An atlas of radiation histopathology. US Energy Research and Administration

28

Ageing

Everybody over 40 is personally aware of the progressive deterioration which we term ageing. Although it is true to say that all bodily functions are affected, some suffer more than others and there is unpredictable variation between individuals. Cerebral degeneration is a frequent symptom of senility with memory, judgement and rational thought often succumbing more than control of movement or sensation. The peculiar sensitivity of nerve cells to anoxia (p. 153) suggests that atheromatous obstruction of blood vessels may be a major factor in ageing of the brain. This may well be the case although neurone loss due to random cell death through cellular senescence is likely to be equally important.

Cardiac function too falls off with advanced age, due partly to reduction in coronary blood flow by atheromatous plaques. The other age-related complications of atheroma have already been discussed (p. 132). With senility there is a reduction in size of the internal organs in general which is due partly to progressive cell loss without replacement and partly to reduction in blood supply.

Some of the most stiking and certainly the most studied aspects of ageing concern the connective tissue. These connective tissue changes are visible in the skin of old people, which becomes dry, wrinkled and inelastic. The events which occur in human skin with advancing age have been characterised in chemical terms. They include a fall in the water content from a high of 86 per cent in the new-born to 60 per cent in old age. Changes occur also in the intercellular matrix of connective tissue which consists of collagen, elastin and proteoglycans. The collagen content of the matrix increases with age especially the insoluble, highly polymerised portion. The turnover rate of collagen is reduced and its half life correspondingly increased. The content of proteoglycans decreases in old age while turnover rate also falls and half life increases. Changes occur in the composition of the glucosaminoglycan component with loss of hyaluronic acid which may account for the dryness of old people's skin since much water is normally bound by this molecule. The content of elastin fibres in skin decreases with age, which with the decline in water accounts for loss of resilience. As the life span of the connective tissue molecules increases with senescence, so the longevity of the cells of skin declines. This is most readily seen in the epidermal cells in which the average life span falls from 100 days in the newborn to 46 days in old age. This situation is aggravated by a parallel fall in the mitotic rate of epidermal epithelium.

Similar changes occur in ageing cartilage, e.g. the articular cartilage of the major joints such as the hip. The alterations in the proportions of collagen and proteoglycans found in senescent skin can be demonstrated equally well in the joint cartilage. The age-dependent chemical changes in proteoglycans have been particularly well documented and include over and under sulphation, hybridisation, increased chain length, altered molecular weight, enlargement of peptide core and changes in amino acid composition. There is a decrease in the cells (chondrocytes) of aged cartilage with a relative increase in older and damaged cells. The chondrocytes show decreased numbers of intracellular organelles especially mitochondria, Golgi vesicles and endoplasmic reticulum. There is an increase in intracellular lipid droplets, phagolysosomes, pigment and fibrils. These complex changes are usually interpreted as indicating diminished cellular metabolism but increased intracellular degradation of collagen and proteoglycans due to age-dependent deterioration in these molecules is also likely. The general degeneration of cartilagenous matrix obviously diminishes the mobility of old people.

Ageing in articular cartilage is hard to differentiate from the disease of osteoarthrosis in which the primary event is degeneration of this cartilage, especially in the hip joint. It may be that the two processes are essentially the same, as osteoarthrosis is almost always a disease of advancing age. Its prominence could be accounted for by the peculiar load-bearing function of the hip joint in man which makes it subject to stresses which are cumulative with age. In joints affected by osteoarthrosis (also known as osteoarthritis) there is depletion of proteoglycans and fragmentation of the collagen fibres. The latter is generally thought to be the primary event and may result from failure due to fatigue like the corresponding event in metals. Probably the contact pressure at the relevant portions of the hip joints are high enough over the age of 50 years to permit fatigue failure to occur.

It is tempting to explain all the manifold changes seen in connective tissue in ageing and osteoarthrosis in terms of fatigue of materials. It should not be forgotten, however, that the materials in question are being destroyed and continually resynthesised by connective tissue cells. The study of chondrocytes in ageing cartilage suggests that the abnormalities of the matrix constituents are due to errors in their synthesis.

The concept of ageing as a cellular process is supported by the limited lifespan of normal cells in tissue culture under optimal conditions. The lifespan of human fibroblasts in ideal cell culture is limited to a mean of about 50 cell divisions per population. Individual cell clones in the population will have shorter or longer life spans due to a capacity for more or less than 50 mitotic divisions. No detectable chromosomal abnormalities are found in association with the shorter life span but fibroblasts from cases of Werner's syndrome, a rare disease of premature ageing associated with chromosomal aberrations have an abnormally brief divisive life span in cell culture.

Paradoxically, cellular ageing can manifest itself as proliferation. This is seen in benign senile prostatic hyperplasia. Presumably as some cells cease to divide, there is failure of negative feed-back and resulting proliferation of the surviving clones. A proliferative stimulus, e.g. platelet factor in atheroma (p. 157) or hormonal imbalance in prostatic hyperplasia (p. 192) will obviously assist division of those cells which still retain the ability to do so.

Two theories are available to explain the ageing of cells. The first, clonal senescence, postulates that the life span of cells is determined by the onset of terminal differentiation, i.e. the point at which in a cell population, all, the cells capable of division (stem cells) disappear and only non-dividing, fully differentiated 'end' cells remain. In a lymph node, lymphocytes would be capable of dividing and plasma cells incapable. In skin, basal epithelium and keratinised squamous cells would be the respective equivalents.

The other theory, now less favoured, is that of error catastrophe. This proposed that one error in transcription or translation during cell division leads to a chain reaction of further errors, culminating in cell death. An example would be synthesis of abnormal cell wall constituents by red corpuscle precursors. This would expose glycoprotein receptors which would bind IgG, which would act as an opsonin and promote phagocytosis of the corpuscles by macrophages. Changes in dividing cells, however, form only part of cellular ageing. Alterations in post-reproductive cells are equally important, as we have already seen in discussing the brain. The ageing of neurones is selective and most cell loss occurs in the locus caeruleus, the superior temporal gyrus, the superior parietal gyrus, the precentral gyrus and the cerebellar purkinje cells. Senescent neurones produce abnormal proteins visible as 'neurofibrillary degeneration' and probably display abnormalities of DNA, RNA and chromosomal proteins.

Ageing of myocardial cells is linked with accumulation of lipofuscin pigment (brown atrophy) due in turn to lipid peroxidation of intracellular membranes. This may be due to senescent inability to produce superoxide dysmutase, which would prevent free O_2^- from wreaking such havoc.

The events of ageing seem unlikely to depend simply on lack of arterial blood due to atheroma and although wear and tear on extracellular materials no doubt plays a part, it is likely that much of the ageing process depends upon cell loss uncompensated by cell division, upon uncorrected errors in the synthesis of cellular constituents and upon diminution in cell metabolism. This inadequacy of function finds many expressions in old age, including not only those we have already mentioned but also growth of facial hair in women, loss of sexual hair and testicular atrophy in men and increased skin pigmentation. The relationship of cancer to ageing is described elsewhere (p. 273).

The progressive deficiency of cell function that we term ageing seems likely to be inherent in the cells themselves if tissue culture experiments are any guide. It is, however, not yet possible to exclude suggestions that the ageing process is controlled by central mechanisms as yet obscure and that these might be influenced by therapy. Cell death occurs in an orderly fashion in all organs throughout our lives and this controlled elimination has special morphological features, the process being known as apoptosis. It is a survival mechanism in the sense that the regulation of the anatomy and function of individual organs depends upon it. As long as reproduction continues, senescence and death of cells remains a survival mechanism and this is true of both individuals and species. Individual survival depends upon appropriate death of cells and their replacement by vigorous successors. Species survival depends upon appropriate death of individuals since environmental resources are finite.

Bibliography

Ali S Y, Elves M W, Leaback D H (eds) 1974 Normal and osteoarthritic articular cartilage. Institue of orthopaedics, University of London

Gaitz C M (ed) 1972 Ageing and the brain. Plenum, New York

Goldstein S 1971 The biology of ageing. New England Journal of Medicine 285: 1120

Martin G M 1977 Cellular ageing. American Journal of Pathology 89: 484

Vogel H G (ed) 1973 Connective tissue and ageing. Excerpta Medica, Amsterdam

29

Hypertrophy, hyperplasia and atrophy

Physiological adaptations to altered bodily needs sometimes become permanent. As an example, if an individual takes phenobarbitone regularly, the microsomal drug-metabolising enzymes of the liver that detoxify the drug become more active and remain so. The ability of microsomal hydroxylases to respond to increased demand by augmented activity is part of the increasing tolerance to drugs which follows their habitual use.

Physiological adaptation which is permanent, or at least sustained for some length of time is frequently accompanied by structural changes, usually an increase in the size of cells (hypertrophy) or an increase in their number (hyperplasia). The best example of physiological hypertrophy is the enlarged skeletal muscles of the athlete or weightlifter. Most examples of physiological hyperplasia are due to the endocrine system working on target organs such as the female breast at puberty, pregnancy, and lactation and the thyroid gland at puberty and pregnancy. In other words, two general mechanisms have evolved which help to adjust to a sustained increased workload on specific organs, an increase in cell size as in muscle subject to augmented exercise, and an increase in cell numbers in an organ responding to endocrine stimulation.

From what we have seen of the parallel evolution of adaptation, and failed adaptation, it would be predicatable that the changes sketched above would have their pathological counterparts and this is indeed the case. The best example of pathological hypertrophy comes from the enlargement of the muscle of the left ventricle of the heart which is a feature of the disease of raised blood pressure. Working against increased pressure, the cardiac muscle cells hypertrophy and for a time their increased size enables cardiac output to be maintained in spite of the extra work-load. Unfortunately, the heart muscle depends for its vigour on the very factor that induced it to enlarge in the first place, i.e. the systemic arterial system which provides its blood supply via the coronary arteries. These vessels do not have an unlimited ability to proliferate in pace with the muscular hypertrophy.

As a result the enlarged heart muscle eventually outstrips its blood supply. In addition, the disease process which started the train of events, i.e. hypertension, leads to accelerated atheroma, especially of the coronary arteries (p. 135). This greatly reduces blood flow through affected vessels. Thus the stimulus for cardiac hypertrophy is also a formula for reducing blood flow to the heart. This means that as the demand of the cardiac muscle for oxygenated blood rises due to its increased cell mass, so its supply of this commodity is progressively reduced. Eventually, therefore, the heart will fail, cardiac output will become inadequate and the patient will die of heart failure unless first carried off by some other result of hypertension such as haemorrhage into the brain.

Hyperplasia too, has many pathological counterparts, although even if understood in general terms the stimulus is seldom identified precisely. A good example is hyperplasia of some of the breast tissues in women causing the disease of cystic hyperplasia. There is an increase in the number of cells in the glands of the breast and in the surrounding connective tissue and some glandular ducts become excessively dilated to form cysts. The nature of the change suggests that it is due to inappropriate and probably excessive hormonal stimulation.

The male counterpart is benign hyperplasia of the prostate gland in which similar changes occur in the glandular tissue. The disease occurs in the elderly and is presumably due to endocrine changes consequent on ageing. The increase in cell numbers may show itself as many normal looking ducts, or as additional cell layers in individual ducts, or as both types of change. The enlarged prostate may block the outflow of urine and cause disease of the renal tract. The increased work involved in voiding urine past an enlarged prostate commonly causes hypertrophy of the muscle in the bladder wall.

Another important example of pathological hyperplasia occurs in the thyroid gland. Here the increase may be diffuse and regular as in Graves' disease, or nodular and irregular as in nodular goitre. Some cases of goitre are due to iodine deficiency but most are of unknown cause. Graves' disease is almost always accompanied by the secretion of abnormally high amounts of thyroid hormone, i.e. by thyrotoxicosis. It is also accompanied by the appearance in the blood of a long acting thyroid stimulating substance (LATS), excessive production of which may be the cause of the disease (p. 55).

All three hyperplastic states described here tend to show concurrent evidence of involution as if periods of increased cellular production were succeeded in irregular cycles by episodes of regression. This accords with the view that they are due to disturbed endocrine control.

The mixed picture of activity and decline has been termed 'dysplasia'. The word is used also to describe abnormal hyperplasia in general as seen for example in the stratified squamous epithelium of the skin in psoriasis. In this instance not only are there more layers of cells than normal but keratin production is disturbed and excessive. In fact, pathological hyperplasia in which tissue architecture appears otherwise normal is unusual although it may occur in endocrine glands, such as the parathyroids, when these are stimulated to increased secretion by disease.

Metaplasia means the transformation of one type of epithelium to another, e.g. a change in the respiratory tract from columnar to squamous cells. This may be important because of concurrent loss of function. In the example quoted, secretion of respiratory mucus is the casualty.

The opposite of hypertrophy and hyperplasia is atrophy and hypoplasia, i.e. a decline in the size of tissues due to diminished numbers of cells or to a reduction in their size. These are physiological events in embryogenesis, infancy and childhood and after pregnancy or the cessation of lactation. In pathology, many circumstances may lead to shrinkage of tissues, notably old age, reduced blood supply (ischaemia), lack of use or endocrine factors.

Bibliography

Bloodworth J M B Jr (ed) 1968 Endocrine pathology. Williams & Wilkins, Baltimore
Ciba Foundation Symposium No. 37 1971 Hypertrophic obstructive cardiomyopathy. Churchill Livingstone, Edinburgh
Stiehl A Thaler M M, Admirand W H 1972 Phenobarbitone and endoplasmic reticulum. New England Journal of Medicine 286: 858

30

Congenital and inherited disease

A congenital disease is one with which the patient is born and an inherited disease is one which is due to factors in the genetic material received from the parents. Both terms are often used loosely or synonymously but an inherited disease might not become apparent until middle age and is not therefore truly congenital. The subject is awesome in scope because quite apart from obvious inherited defects, and these are numerous enough, even infectious diseases, such as tuberculosis, may exhibit inherited susceptibility as may conditions as diverse as cancer (p. 264) or cardiac infarction (p. 135). The bulk of this chapter, however, will concern itself with diseases in which intrauterine or inherited factors are the sole or major determining element. For simplicity also I will use congenital to include all diseases inherited or acquired in utero.

In dealing with so large a subject some form of classification becomes a necessity rather than a pedantic exercise. This is because even to a layman, congenital disease involves disabilities as various as anatomical malformations, such as septal defects of the heart, mental subnormality, functional defects such as haemophilia or tragic sequalae to inadvertent poisoning of the fetus as with thalidomide.

The physician who sees congenital disease also feels baffled by the complexities of the subject, especially the permutations of different anatomical deformities appearing sometimes singly, sometimes together, with or without mental subnormality. At the same time he wishes to correlate the abnormalities he observes in the patient with the information fed to him by contemporary genetics. These physicians have therefore put forward a suggested classification of congenital disease as follows:

1. **Specific syndromes**
   A. *Known cause*
      Major gene defects
      (i) known chemical defect
      (ii) unknown chemical defect
      Chromosomal abnormalities

Major environmental factor
Multifactoral
  B. *Unknown causes*
2. *Provisional syndromes or associations*
3. *Anomalies* (a single localised anatomical anomaly in early morphogenesis)

This classification will be helpful to those attempting to identify specific disease syndromes but is unsatisfactory to the pathologist because it fits uneasily with genetics and cell biology, being based partly on causes and partly on effects. On the other hand a detailed aetiological classification is not yet possible. For the purposes of this chapter therefore it is proposed to consider congenital disease as falling into one of three categories as follows:

1. Abnormalities of genes
2. Abnormalities of chromosomes
3. Polygenic inheritance + abnormalities occurring after fertilisation.

This classification is based not so much on aetiology as on pathogenesis since a variety of factors known or unknown could activate any of these mechanisms.

Before discussing this important topic it is necessary briefly to review current knowledge of inheritance and intrauterine development. This involves two separate subjects; the transmission of genetic information (genetics) and the control of growth and differentiation in the developing embryo (embryology). The pathological counterpart of embryology is teratology, the scientific study of congenital malformations. Since morphological defects present at birth may be monogenic, polygenic or environmental, teratology can involve study of all these mechanisms.

For the purposes of this chapter there are two types of cell, somatic or body cells and germ cells, i.e. ova or sperm. The information needed to reproduce a replica of a somatic cell is contained in the chromosomes of its nucleus. These can be studied by arresting the cell in the metaphase stage of mitotic division. The chromosomes can be stained by a variety of techniques, photographed and arranged in order of size and shape.

A somatic cell contains 46 chromosomes consisting of 44 somatic or autosomal chromosomes (autosomes) and 2 sex chromosomes. The autosomes consist of 22 pairs each pair consisting of two identical partners and differing in size and configuration from all the other 21 pairs. In females the sex chromosomes consist of 2 apparently identical

X-chromosomes; in males of an X and a Y chromosome, quite different in size and shape. To assist mapping, chromosomes are numbered according to the Denver classification in decreasing order of size so that chromosome pair number 1 is the largest and pair 22 the smallest. The sex chromosomes X and Y are not numbered. Special stains, e.g. quinacrine mustard induce bright fluorescence under UV light in the Y chromosome which helps its identification. The X chromosome can be seen in nondividing female cells as a dark spot on the inner surface of the nuclear membrane (Barr body) or as a drum-stick-shaped nodule in the nuclei of female leucocytes. In addition to numbering the chromosomes they can be grouped more simply, again according to size and shape. In the agreed Denver-London system; group A includes chromosomes 1 to 3; group B numbers 4 and 5; group C, 6 to 12 plus the X chromosome or chromosomes; group D, 13 to 15; group E, 16 to 18; group F, 19 and 20 and group G, 21 and 22 plus the Y chromosome. The classification of chromosomes is an essential preliminary to understanding congenital disease due to chromosomal defects.

When a somatic cell divides, the chromosomes first double in number to 92. As mitosis is completed (anaphase) half of these go to each daughter cell which now has its normal complement of 46. New animals and people are formed by fusion of a gamete from one individual with the gamete from another. To produce off-spring with 46 chromosomes it is essential therefore that each gamete contains only 23 chromosomes. This is achieved in the ovaries and testes respectively, by the gamete precursor cells undergoing a special form of division (meiosis) in which the number of chromosomes is halved. In effect, the precursor cell divides into two gametes without first doubling the number of its chromosomes. Since the chromosomes in the precursor cell (as in all cells other than gametes) are duplicated in identical pairs, it is necessary only for each pair to separate in order to form perfect gametes containing all the needed genetic information, although in the case of male gametes, half will have the X chromosome and half the Y chromosome.

The chromosomes carry genetic information because each is a long strand of DNA consisting of numerous genes strung together on the chromosome like a rope of pearls. A gene (also called a cistron) is a strand of DNA and the unit of genetic transcription because it codes usually for one protein. It is composed of many sub-units called codons, each codon consisting of a triplet of nucleotides from one strand of DNA. Each triplet codes for one amino acid with the assistance of the messenger RNA (mRNA) containing the complementary sequence of bases.

DNA consists of pentose sugar, phosphate and combinations of four bases, cytosine (C), thymine (T), adenine (A) and guanine (G). It is the bases which confer individuality to genes. Each pair of bases links two strands of the sugar-phosphate components. Only four kinds of base pairings are possible, AT, TA, CG and GC. Each gene consists of about 1500 base pairs arranged with the attached pentose and phosphate in the famous double helix. As we have said, three successive base pairs form a codon. Because three base pairs is the smallest unit possible and because only four types of base pair are possible there are 64 possible triplet codons (i.e. 4^3). This would allow up to 64 amino acids to be formed (in fact there are about 20). Some codons have other functions such as signalling the beginning or end of transcription. Finally, it will be appreciated that the time-honoured concept of one gene—one protein (or enzyme) is valid in the sense that there are about 500 codons in a gene (cistron) and about 500 amino acids in an average protein and each codon determines one amino acid. Haemoglobin has two proteins, alpha and beta, each with its own gene. However, some complex proteins or even groups of proteins (e.g. the enzymes involved in the metabolism of histidine) have their production controlled by one giant gene (polycistron) collaborating with a specially long mRNA.

The way in which DNA in the form of structural genes induces the formation of cellular products and structures via messenger RNA and transfer RNA (tRNA) is not really relevant to congenital disease. However, messenger RNA like DNA is formed in the nucleus and the formation of both is under the control of operator genes which switches it on and off. Thus a liver cell has the inherent capacity to make thyroid gland hormone but does not do so because the operator gene in the liver cell has switched off the structural gene which in the thyroid cell codes for that particular protein. It is obvious that since all cells contain all the chromosomes and all the genetic data for the whole organism, in any given cell very many structural genes must be in the switched-off position. The operator genes are themselves controlled by regulator genes which are responsive to environmental changes and act by way of repressor proteins. One operator gene often controls many individual structural genes, e.g. the polycistron responsible for histidine metabolism mentioned above.

In inherited disease the system fails not at this stage but at a point where the DNA molecule replicates itself during cell division by acquiring new bases from the nuclear sap to form new base pairs. If mistakes occur, faulty base pairing results and leads to mutation. Figure 30.1 shows the normal process of DNA replication as it occurs in dividing cells. The process has been likened by Roberts to the

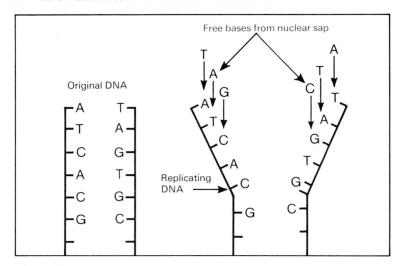

Fig. 30.1 One way in which single gene abnormalities originate. At the time of mitotic DNA replication in the germ cell, if new bases from the nuclear sap pair up in the wrong order the new DNA is not an accurate copy of the original and a point mutation occurs.

formation of two new zip fasteners from one. As new bases arrive, the original paired strands of DNA peel away from each other carrying the newly attached bases with them. Mutation can occur at the level of individual genes (point mutation) or can involve whole chromosomes. In both cases it usually happens when the DNA strand is dividing and can occur spontaneously or be induced by ionising radiation or chemicals.

The steps we have so far considered lead to the formation of gametes which may produce normal off-spring or may yield children with an inherited defect due to faulty genetic or chromosomal behaviour. Defective fertilisation of the gamete or faulty implantation in the uterus of the fertilised ovum may abort the conception but are unlikely to lead to congenital disease. Abnormal development of the embryo after successful fertilisation and implantation is, however, a major cause of such illness. Unfortunately, compared with the mass of information on genetics, there is a great deal of ignorance concerning the environmental factors controlling growth and development of the fetus.

Bibliography for Chapter 30 appears on p. 219

31

Genetically determined diseases

These are conditions which can be traced in family trees and which are inherited according to the principles of Mendelian genetics. This means that they are due to point mutations in single genes and called monogenic. From the viewpoint of the geneticist they come in three types, dominant, intermediate or recessive. From the viewpoint of the pathologist they are manifest in two ways; as anatomical defects, obvious grossly at birth or as abnormalities, functional or structural or both, which become apparent during childhood or adult life. In this latter group come the classical inborn errors of metabolism in which the abnormality, however wide-reaching its effects, can often be traced to lack of a single enzyme. Also in the group is the much studied disease of haemophilia due to deficiency of a particular protein. Another disease in the group, which because of the painting by Velasquez is as famous as haemophilia, is achondroplasia, a characteristic growth defect. In achondroplasia as in other genetically determined anatomical disorders, the widespread structural abnormalities are probably determined by a relatively simple but as yet unknown biochemical defect.

When a single protein or enzyme is demonstrably deficient, as in haemophilia or phenylketonuria, an error in coding has occurred involving a single gene or cistron, since this is the genetic unit responsible for a single protein. In fact, the error may be restricted to one codon since only one amino acid in the protein may be wrongly placed, as it is in the abnormal haemoglobin which when inherited causes the disease of sickle cell anaemia. To the molecular and cellular biologist, the interest of genetic disease lies in the particular segments of the DNA strands which are wrongly assembled so that they code for an abnormal protein. As we have noted earlier these errors occur during the replication of the DNA strands (chromosomes), are due to faulty pairing of bases and are known as mutations. Mutations can be caused by irradiation or by chemicals or drugs or can occur spontaneously. Some genes are especially liable to spontaneous mutation.

These unstable cistrons include those responsible for two diseases already mentioned, haemophilia and achondroplasia.

A chart of the inborn errors of metabolism, prepared by B. E. Nicholson, shows about 70 such diseases, each due to a genetically determined deficiency of one particular enzyme. The enzyme may be present in the mitochondria, endoplasmic reticulum, or lysosomes and no aspect of metabolism is spared. One of the most important consequences of these metabolic defects is mental subnormality, the brain cells being especially susceptible to damage from abnormal chemical metabolites. Mental impairment can develop from very different causes ranging from the abnormal accumulation of intracellular lipids due to lack of a lysosomal enzyme, sphingomyelinase (Niemann-Pick's disease) to the accumulation of a toxic metabolite of phenylalanine due to lack of phenylalanine hydroxylase (phenylketonuria). These metabolic errors affect the child at a crucial stage of its development and if it can be tided over by feeding artificial diets free of the substrate, e.g. phenylalanine which yields the toxic products, it may in adult life be found to have enough of the appropriate enzyme to live normally.

The examples of genetic disease so far quoted are easy enough to understand on the basis of errors of coding in specific cistrons or codons. However, there are conditions which are passed on from one generation to the next in classical Mendelian fashion but in which it is more difficult to imagine the mode of action of the faulty gene. There is for example the disease of anonychia in which there is a variable degree of malformation of the hands or nails. If the development of individual parts of the body were controlled directly by individual genes, there should be many other examples of comparable malformations inherited by Mendelian laws, but there are not. It may be therefore that in anonychia there is deficiency of a particular bodily protein or enzyme the lack of which is critical only as regards the hands and nails. Similarly, some forms of cancer are transmitted by genetic faults, e.g. neuroblastoma or polyposis coli and there are strange and rare families in which thickening of the soles of the feet and cancer of the oesophagus are inherited in classical Mendelian fashion. It is difficult to make such pedigrees fit the accepted facts of gene action, but not impossible, since a single protein or enzyme could be imagined which restrains uncontrolled growth of certain cells or which inactivates certain cancer-inducing metabolites.

These are mere hypotheses, however, and they show that genetically determined diseases cannot be explained easily by contemporary molecular biology unless they can be pinned down to a deficiency or abnormality of one particular protein. We can predict, nevertheless, that in many examples now obscure, an underlying biochemical lesion will be found.

In the meantime, the known genetic abnormalities provide a rich spectrum of disease mechanisms. The haemoglobin gene seems especially vulnerable and there are many diseases associated with abnormal haemoglobin. The best known of these is sickle-cell anaemia in which although only one amino acid is wrongly placed, fatal haemolytic anaemia may result due to crystallisation of haemoglobin and disruption of red blood corpuscles. There are many other types of haemolytic anaemia due to deficiencies of various respiratory enzymes in the red cell, e.g. glucose-6-P-dehydrogenase. There are a variety of disorders of carbohydrate metabolism due to deficiency of a single sugar-metabolising enzyme, e.g. galactose-1-P-uridyl transferase which causes the disease galactosaemia, resulting in mental subnormality and death. Glycogen may be stored in vast amounts in liver or spleen due to lack of one of eight glycogen-metabolising enzymes. There are similar storage diseases of lipids, e.g. Gauchers disease due to genetically determined deficiency of glucosyl-cerebroside hydrolase (glucoceribrosidase). The porphyrin metabolising enzymes may be absent with catastrophic results (George III is reputed to have suffered from one disease in this category and the loss of the American colonies has been blamed on his porphyria). Amino acid metabolising enzymes may be deficient, e.g. tyrosinase leading to the albino state (melanin pigment cannot be formed) or phenylalanine hydroxylase causing phenylketonuria and mental defect as already mentioned. Purine or pyrimidine metabolism may be disturbed, e.g. due to lack of xanthine oxidase, leading to xanthinuria so that stones form in the kidney. Gout is another inherited and much more common disorder of purine metabolism. This list is very far from complete but should give some idea of the scope of the subject even though many of these diseases are extremely rare.

Dominant inheritance

In this situation every individual carrying the abnormal gene suffers from the disease. Most serious genetic diseases are not dominant for the simple reason that a serious dominant genetic defect would soon extinguish itself from the population unless loss of a gene through death or infertility of the affected individual were balanced by a corresponding high mutation rate. This is the state of affairs in achondroplasia, which is due to defective metabolism in bone epiphyses. The mutation rate of this dominant gene has been measured and found to be 1 : 20 000. This means that once in every 20 000 replications the normal gene mutates. Since every individual has two such genes, one on each of the chromosome pair, he has two chances of suffering mutation, so that one child in 10 000 suffers from achondroplasia due to mutation in a parental gene. The achondroplastic population appears to be fairly constant in size, in spite of the fact that up to 80 per cent die during childhood, which means that the rate of elimination due to the lowered average reproductive rate of those carrying the gene is balanced by the high mutation rate. In fact, the mutation rate can be calculated by equating it to the average effective fertility of affected persons as compared with normals. Dominant genes are controlled by the mutation rate for that gene. If reproduction is nil the gene can only be perpetuated by a very high mutation rate.

A dominant gene can be regarded as a defect a single dose of which is able to produce disease. Thus most affected persons are heterozygous, i.e. one of the pair of genes is normal and the other is the abnormal mutant. There are rare cases in which an achondroplastic was found to be homozygous for the trait, i.e. both genes were abnormal, which means that he had received an achondroplastic gene from both parents. This double dose of defective genetic material produced an achondroplastic not obviously different from a heterozygous achondroplastic. In the case of other dominant abnormal genes this is not the case. Thus those homozygous for brachydactyly (short fingers) have severe, widespread skeletal defects, whereas the heterozygotes merely have short fingers.

Recessive inheritance

A genetic abnormality is inherited recessively if it expresses itself only when present on both members of the affected chromosome pair of the individual concerned (Fig. 31.1). In other words a double dose of the abnormal gene is required to produce the disease. A single dose, i.e. one abnormal gene, produces no effect because it is dominated and suppressed by the corresponding normal gene on the other chromosome. This is the only difference between dominant and recessive genes but their distribution in the population is very different.

For any particular abnormal gene, heterozygotes are much more common than homozygotes (Fig. 31.2). Thus albinism (due to a defect in genetic coding for tyrosinase) affects about 1 in 10 000 people. Any given person stands a 1 in a 100 chance of receiving the abnormal gene on one of the relevant chromosome pair and a 1 in a 100 chance of receiving it on the other chromosome of the pair and therefore a 1 in 50 chance of receiving it on one or other chromosome. This means that 1 person in 50 will be heterozygous for albinism. However, the chance of receiving two albinism genes, i.e. one from each parent, is 1 in 100×1 in 100, i.e. 1 in 10 000 which is the risk of being an albino.

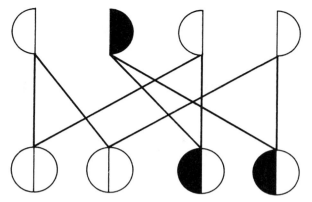

Fig. 31.1 Mendelian inheritance of disease. The semi circles represent the parental gametes. The dark gametes carry the abnormal gene. The full circles represent the offspring. In this illustration one parent is heterozygous for the abnormal gene; the other parent is normal. Half the offspring will have the abnormal gene: if it is recessive, they will not develop the disease; if it is dominant they will do so.

When we see that a frequency of heterozygotes of 1 in 50 is necessary to produce 1 in 10 000 affected individuals, we realise how common are the genes of recessively inherited diseases compared with the diseases themselves, and how easily an abnormal recessive gene can be passed on undetected through several generations. Affected individuals usually arise from the mating of unaffected parents each of whom, however, is heterozygous for the condition. They will produce one affected (homozygous) child for every three unaffected (heterozygous) children. Since an individual carrying a defective gene is more likely to

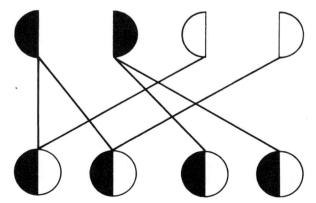

Fig. 31.2 In this example, one parent is homozygous for the above gene and one parent is normal—all offspring carry the affected gene.

encounter that gene within his own family than in the general population, consanguinous marriages, e.g. between first cousins, have a
greater than average chance of producing a homozygous, i.e. affected

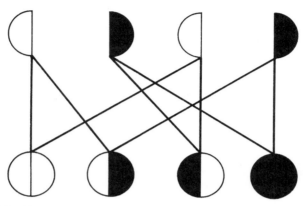

Fig. 31.3 In this example, both parents are heterozygous. Three children out of
four will inherit the gene and one of them will be homozygous and develop the
disease even if it is recessive.

child (Fig. 31.3). Consanguinous marriage does not influence the
dominant gene inheritance of diseases such as achondroplasia where a
single dose of defective gene material is sufficient.

Intermediate inheritance
We have seen that rare individuals who are homozygous for some
dominant genes have a more severe form of disease than the more
usual heterozygotes. Conversely, some heterozygotes with recessive
genes show a milder form of the disturbance displayed by those with
both defective genes, i.e. the homozygotes. This incomplete expression in heterozygotes is known as intermediate inheritance and is of
importance in tracing carriers of a defective gene. There are several
important examples of intermediate inheritance in human pathology.
The gene of phenylketonuria is revealed in carriers, i.e. heterozygotes
not suffering from the disease, by biochemical tests which show
impaired breakdown of phenylalanine. The same is true of galactosaemia. In sickle-cell anaemia, disease-free heterozygotes carrying
only one sickle cell gene exhibit the so called sickle-cell trait. This
means that their red cells are healthy in normal circumstances but
become fragile if exposed to a high CO_2 concentration in a test tube. A
somewhat similar situation exists in another genetically determined
haemolytic anaemia known as thalassaemia. The heterozygotes are

said to have thalassaemia minor and the homozygotes, thalassaemia major.

Sex-linked inheritance

If a mutant gene happens to be sited on the X or Y chromosomes the chance of an individual being affected will depend upon his or her sex. In practice, the X chromosome is usually involved because it contains about 80 possible mutant genes, including haemophilia, colour blindness and muscular dystrophy (Table 31.1). The male has only one X chromosome, so dominance and recessivity do not arise since there is no corresponding gene (allele) on the other chromosome to suppress or be suppressed, the other half of the chromosome pair being the Y chromosome. Hence, if a male carries the mutant gene he will exhibit the disease. If a female carries the mutant gene, she may or may not be affected depending on whether the gene is dominant or recessive and whether she is homozygous or heterozygous, i.e. whether she has inherited a single or double dose of aberrant genetic material. Thus, all males who inherit the haemophilia gene on their single X chromosome (1 in 10000 males) will have haemophilia, but female haemophiliacs will be confined to those who inherit the gene on both their X chromosomes, an exceedingly rare event. In other words, although haemophilia is carried on the female chromosome, practically all haemophiliacs are male. The chances of a female being a haemophiliac are 1 in 100 million, i.e. 1 in 10000×1 in 10000.

The 'Simple Equation'

It is not necessary to go through professional life committing to memory those disorders which are dominant and those which are recessive. It is easier to remember the simple equation which states that in general, dominant diseases are caused by mutations in genes coding for structural proteins (not to be confused with structural genes—something quite different) and that recessive diseases are caused by mutations in genes coding for enzymes.

In fact it is not even necessary to remember the equation, only to understand its obvious reason. This is that enzymes have a big margin for error, so that the recessive heterozygote patient although having only half the normal enzyme (and half the abnormal) nevertheless does not manifest disease. On the other hand in dominant conditions, heterozygotes develop the disease because with structural proteins there is little margin for error. If half the structure is normal and half abnormal it will be too weak to function.

The haemoglobinopathies are recessive, but haemoglobin, being a carrier molecule, is as much an enzyme as a structural protein. Some

Table 31.1 Mode of inheritance of some genetic diseases

Dominant	Recessive	Intermediate	Sex linked (X chromosome)	Sex linked (Y chromosome)
Achondroplasia	Fibrocystic disease of the pancreas	Thalassaemia major/minor	Haemophilia	Hairy ears
Polyposis coli	Phenylketonuria	Sickle cell anaemia/trait	Muscular dystrophy (Duchenne type)	
Huntingdon's chorea	Albinism		Colour Blindness	
Epiloia	Galactosaemia		Chronic granulomatous disease	
Porphyria variegata	Muscular dystrophy (late onset type)			
Retinal aplasia	Cretinism			
Anonychia	Lipid storage diseases			
Congenital cataract	Carbohydrate storage diseases			
Marfan's syndrome	Glucose-6-phosphate–Dehydrogenase deficiency			
	Most other inborn errors of metabolism			

other seeming exceptions in which enzyme deficiencies appear to be dominant are due to primary defects in structural proteins controlling the enzyme, e.g. cell membrane components, or to an excess of enzyme inhibitor.

A source of confusion is the occurrence of the same disease in both dominant and recessive forms. One example is the Ehlers-Danlos syndrome, a disorder of connective tissue. Here the recessive varieties are due to defects in the enzymes involved in collagen synthesis. The dominant types of the syndrome have no demonstrable enzyme deficiency and are probably due to structural abnormalities in collagen itself.

Genetic disease and natural selection

In this book we have encountered several examples of pathology arising as a by-product of an evolutionary survival mechanism. The basis of genetic disease is harmful mutation which then persists in the population. This persistence may seem hard to understand because affected individuals should slowly be eliminated by natural selection. It is important to realise, however, that the human race is apparently committed to continuing evolution and that this can only be achieved by the process of mutation that we have described. Obviously therefore some of these mutations will be harmful and others beneficial. With regard to persistence of harmful genes, we have to realise that we do not always see the whole picture. The sickle-cell trait described above is extremely common in some parts of the world, notably Africa, where 20 to 30 per cent of the population may have the gene. Such prevalence suggests a survival advantage in heterozygotes which outweighs the death rate from sickle-cell anaemia in the homozygotes. In fact, the abnormal gene confers a great deal of protection against malaria, since the abnormal red cells do not support the malarial parasite as efficiently as normal corpuscles. As malaria is one of the commonest causes of death in children and people of reproductive age in these regions, the sickle cell gene has strong survival value and persists through natural selection. When the Africans move to countries where malaria is not endemic, the gene loses its value and slowly disappears, as a result of natural selection eliminating the homozygotes. This process is going on in the black population of the USA and provides an example of Darwinism in action. An interesting although less well documented example of the survival value of disease-causing genetic mutation is the decreased susceptibility to tuberculosis associated with the lysosomal storage diseases with their epicentre in Eastern Europe. These include Gauchers, Tay-Sachs and Niemann-Pick disease.

When a mutation first occurs, the mutant gene is at first neither dominant nor recessive. If the change is favourable for the species concerned, dominance will develop due to natural selection favouring a weak corresponding gene on the other chromosome of the pair (the allele, in genetic terminology). If the mutation is unfavourable when fully expressed it will become recessive due to natural selection promoting a strong suppressive unmutated gene on the other chromosome. It follows from this that once a gene has become dominant, provided it does not prevent reproduction, it is no longer subject to the pressures of natural selection, whereas a recessive gene is always at risk of disappearing. We have seen why some common recessive genes such as that of sickle-cell anaemia persist but in other cases, for example cystic fibrosis of the pancreas, there is no apparent reason. Achondroplasia (dominant) and haemophilia (recessive) seem to remain in the population because of the very high spontaneous mutation rate of the genes concerned.

Polygenic inheritance as a contributing factor in disease

Thus far we have considered only diseases wholly determined by specific mutant genes. There is, however, good evidence that many other diseases, caused by a multiplicity of factors, have a familial component. Essential hypertension is an important and common disease in which the arterial blood pressure is abnormally high for no apparent reason. The level of blood pressure in the population follows the usual Gaussian distribution pattern with most people having normal blood pressure, some having lower than average pressure and some having higher than average. This latter group is said to have essential hypertension and although some may remain symptom free, many others will suffer fatal consequences such as cerebral haemorrhage or heart failure. For any given level of blood pressure there is a tendency of first degree relatives, i.e. parents, off-spring and siblings to resemble each other with respect to blood pressure. This tendency is of a similar order for all first degree relatives and the genetic element in determining blood pressure is therefore not of Mendelian type.

In duodenal ulcer, 8 per cent of the brothers of ulcer patients also have ulcers whereas the expected figure had there been no familial tendency would have been 3 per cent. There is no evidence to suggest transmission by a single gene.

In cancer, single gene inheritance occurs only in one or two specific instances, e.g. neuroblastoma and polyposis coli. In most cases, however, where a familial trend can be shown at all it is of the type described above as occurring in duodenal ulceration.

These instances are probably examples of polygenic inheritance. This means that some individuals inherit a general genetic package which predisposes them to certain illnesses and renders them susceptible to certain environmental influences, mostly of unknown nature. The concept is supported by certain statistical observations such as that people with blood group O are 40 per cent more likely to develop a duodenal ulcer than those with other blood groups. Blood group and tissue transplantation antigens are inherited in mendelian fashion but seem sometimes to act as markers for the polygenic transmission of susceptibility to certain diseases. The HLA system is a special example of this and because of its importance is dealt with in a separate section (p. 220).

Bibliography for Chapter 31 appears on p. 219.

32

Chromosomal abnormalities

Genes are molecules of DNA and genetic defects occur therefore at the molecular level. Chromosomes are strands of genetic material large enough to be seen with the light microscope and chromosomal abnormalities are by definition visible by light microscopy.

Defects of single genes may cause fatal disease, so it is not surprising that chromosomal aberrations involving hundreds or thousands of genes are usually incompatible with life. The only situation in which an entire chromosome may be absent and the individual survive is in females who lack one of their X chromosomes (see below). Major deficiency of even part of a somatic chromosome is rarely compatible with survival and occurs only in some very uncommon disorders of childhood.

These remarks of course apply to situations in which the chromosomal abnormality is present in all the cells of the body. Particular cell populations, especially malignant tumours (p. 242) or inflammatory macrophages (Fig. 32.1) may show gross disturbances of chromosome

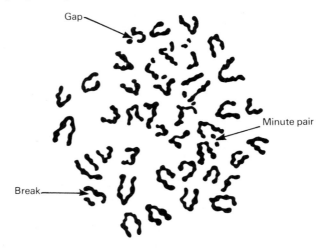

Fig. 32.1 Gross chromosomal abnormalities in an inflammatory macrophage.

pattern but if the tumour is eradicated, and the macrophages eliminated (p. 122), the patient's survival will not be affected.

With the exceptions mentioned, chromosomal mutations as defined above, i.e. visible by light microscopy, affecting all somatic cells and compatible with life, occur usually in the form of an additional whole chromosome.

Chromosomes are studied by allowing cells from bone marrow or skin to divide in culture, arresting mitosis in metaphase and then inducing the chromosomes to spread out. The maps obtained in this way are known as karyotypes and the chromosomes classified and numbered (p. 196).

The detection of chromosomal abnormalities has been greatly improved by the use of banding techniques. These are special stains which pick out the chromosome very clearly. Band staining can be achieved with Giemsa (G), Chloroquine (C), reverse staining (R) or Chromatin staining (C). These stains delineate different regions and bands on the chromosome so it is necessary to specify which was used. Using all possible permutations, up to 10 000 bands can be detected on human chromosomes, if special techniques are used which 'stretch' the chromosome. As a result of these advances, 30 new chromosomal syndromes have been described in the past few years. Most of the new defects can be localised quite specifically, e.g. deletion of band 2 in region 14 of the long arm of chromosome 13 in retinoblastoma, a malignant tumour of childhood. This is written 13q14.2. If the short arm of the chromosome is affected the letter p is substituted for q.

Chromosomal abnormalities are much more common than genetic mutations. About 4 per cent of newly conceived human fetuses have chromosomal aberrations and of these abnormal conceptuses about 90 per cent will be aborted in the early months of pregnancy. Of abortions occurring spontaneously early in pregnancy 20 to 40 per cent exhibit and presumably result from incorrect chromosomal patterns. Absence of one X chromosome is a common cause of non-viability, especially in male fetuses.

Some of the best studied chromosomal disturbances affect the sex chromosomes. The abnormalities are due to non-disjunction at the stage of meiosis when DNA strands separate to form the gametes (p. 196) (Fig. 32.2). This means that a chromosome pair fails to separate and that as a result the gametes will contain either both sex chromosomes or neither. The sperm of a male parent showing non-disjunction will contain either an X plus a Y chromosome, two X's or two Y's or no sex chromosomes at all. A female similarly affected will produce ova with two X chromosomes or no sex chromosomes (Fig. 32.3). Using the analogy of the zip fastener (p. 198) non-disjunction represents a

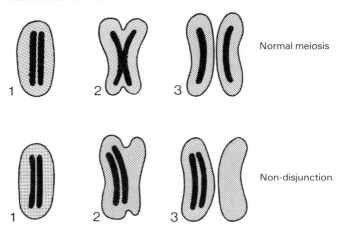

Fig. 32.2 Non-disjunction of chromosomes at meiosis.

failure of the unzipping process with both halves of the fastener coming away together from the cloth to which it was sewn. The permutations of sex chromosomes possible in the off-spring of gametes showing non-disjunction are best understood by studying the accompanying table (Table 32.1).

Super-females and super-males, disappointingly differ little from normal, but Klinefelter's syndrome cases exhibit small testes, subfertility and possibly other defects although usually outwardly normal.

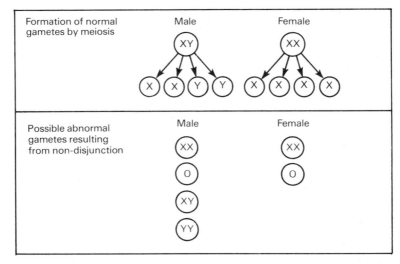

Fig. 32.3 The formation of abnormal sex gametes as a result of non-disjunction.

Table 32.1 Some sexual abnormalities resulting from chromosomal nondisjunction

Gametes		Offspring	Clinical state
Ova normal	Sperm abnormal		
X	XY	XXY	Klinefelter's syndrome
X	XX	XXX	Super-female
X	YY	XYY	Super-male
X	O	XO	Turner's syndrome
Ova abnormal	Sperm normal		
XX	Y	XXY	Klinefelter's syndrome
XX	X	XXX	Super-female
O	X	XO	Turner's syndrome
O	Y	OY	Non-viable

Turner's syndrome patients are phenotypically female i.e. look like women, but the external genitalia are small and the ovaries are mere rudiments. Many other abnormalities may be present, e.g. small stature, webbing of the neck, deafness or cardiac abnormalities.

About one male in 500 has Klinefelter's syndrome, one female in 2500 Turner's syndrome and one female in 1250 has the XXX genotype. With regard to Turner's syndrome, i.e. the XO genotype, (table 32.1) since 97 per cent of these are aborted in the fetal stage, about 0.8 per cent, almost 1 in 100 of all conceptions have this chromosomal aberration. Many other anomalies of the X chromosome are known in which additional X chromosomes are present. As a result there has been wide acceptance of the hypothesis advanced by Dr Lyon which in its simplified form states that only one X chromosome remains active in any cell. It appears also that the Y chromosome is very powerful since individuals with two, three or even four X chromosomes and one Y chromosome are apparently normal males although usually subfertile.

Most states of intersexuality are due to causes other than chromosomal abnormalities. True hermaphrodites i.e. with gonads of both sexes have either a normal XX genotype (50 per cent) or a normal XY genotype (20 per cent). The remaining 30 per cent have XX karyotypes in some of their cells and XY karyotypes in others. This is known as mosaicism and is an important aspect of medical genetics but is beyond the scope of this book.

Down's syndrome (mongolism)

At least 1 in 600 live births suffers from this condition. It is due to an aberration in the autosomes as opposed to the sex chromosomes and consists of an extra chromosome corresponding in size to the 21 or 22 pair but in practice always referred to as 21. Patients with Down's syndrome therefore have 47 chromosomes and are said to exhibit trisomy 21, i.e. 3 autosomes of no. 21 type (Fig. 32.4). The karyotype of a female mongol would be written by a geneticist as 47 XX 21 +, i.e. 47 chromosomes; XX sexual genotype; an extra no. 21 chromosome.

The main manifestation of Down's syndrome is mental subnormality, often severe. This is associated with various physical abnormalities including the heavy folds of skin over the corners of the eyes which led to the term mongolism. More serious physical defects include congenital heart disease and a tendency to develop leukaemia. The main cause of mongolism is non disjunction of the 21 chromosome pair at meiosis, so that some gametes contain 2 of these chromosomes instead of 1, (Fig. 32.5). There is a very striking tendency for this to become more frequent with an increase in the age of the mother. In mothers under 30 years old the incidence is 1 in 2250 live births. In mothers aged 35 to 40 years the incidence is 1 in 200. If a mongol has an identical twin it will almost certainly be affected but only 1 in 100 of the siblings is likely to be a mongol. These facts are what would be expected in a

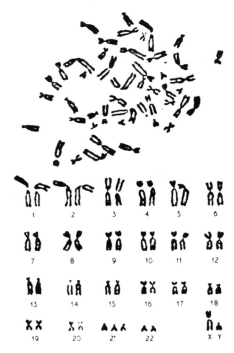

Fig. 32.4 The karyotype of a male child with Down's syndrome showing three no. 21 chromosomes.

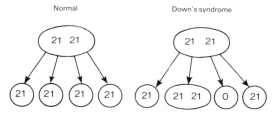

Fig. 32.5 Non-disjunction of chromosome 21 causing Down's syndrome.

disease due to chromosomal abnormality in the germ cell. Presumably non-disjunction is an event the probability of which increases dramatically with maternal age. In addition to mongolism, other clinical syndromes of mental and physical abnormality are known, associated with trisomy of chromosomes other than number 21.

Down's syndrome can also appear in children who seem to have the normal number of chromosomes. In these the extra 21 chromosome is present but fused to another chromosome, e.g. no. 14, forming a giant composite chromosome. The mothers of such children have one less than the normal number of chromosomes because one of their no. 21 pair also is fused to another. This fusion is known as translocation and like non-disjunction occurs during meiosis. It has no association with maternal age but can be passed on through the generations so that apparently normal carriers produce mongol children. With mothers under 30 years, about 10 per cent of mongol children are due to translocation and 90 per cent to non-disjunction. With mothers over 30 years of age the figures are 1 per cent and 99 per cent respectively.

The rare group of congenital diseases due to absence of chromosomal material are often associated with deletion of part of chromosome no. 6 and present as a variety of clinical syndromes. Chromosomal deletion, like non-disjunction and translocation takes place during meiosis. Many of the features of Down's syndrome occur in other less common chromosomal abnormalities. Mongoloid, slanting eyes occur in 12 defects other than trisomy 21, congenital heart disease in 22 types & mental retardation in 36. The reasons for these curious propensities, which also include transverse palmar creases, are mysterious.

The way in which chromosomal aberrations cause abnormalities is less clear than in the case of point mutations involving single genes where a biochemical explanation is available. Presumably a quantitative disturbance in the distribution of chromatin upsets the balance of genetic material and interferes with the expression of single major genes or multiple minor genes.

Bibliography for chapter 32 appears on p. 219.

33

Congenital malformations, polygenic inheritance and the fetal environment

The preceding three chapters have said little about the most common congenital diseases, which are anatomical malformations affecting the heart and great vessels, the gastrointestinal and urinary tracts and the skeletal and central nervous systems. Unfortunately less is known about the causation of these deformities than about the conditions already dealt with, most of which are of much smaller importance in clinical medicine. The overall incidence of congenital malformations in Great Britain is about 16 per 1000 total births.

It is generally accepted that very few cases of congenital anatomical defects exhibit the classical Mendelian ratios that would be demonstrable if single gene inheritance were involved. In addition a small minority form part of the clinical pattern associated with particular chromosomal abnormalities e.g. congenital heart disease in trisomy 21 or cleft palate in trisomy 13(p. 215). On the other hand there is a slow accumulation of evidence to indicate that in a surprisingly high number of cases of such anatomical anomalies a definite but less obvious familial tendency is apparent. This tendency is of the type that geneticists associate with polygenic inheritance (p. 208). This means that in any thousand families there is a continuous variation in the likelihood of producing a child with a defect such as congenital heart disease. This likelihood will follow a Gaussian distribution pattern with low, medium and high incidences comparable with the chances of producing short, medium or tall offspring. A pattern of continuous variation in the population is one feature of polygenic inheritance. Another is the tendency for first degree relatives, i.e. parents and siblings all to be 'half-like' each other. This contrasts with single gene classical Mendelian inheritance in which half might be totally like and half totally unlike.

Polygenic inheritance appears to be due to the additive effect of a large number of genes of small effect whereas the effects of single gene inheritance are due to the single action of a gene of large effect. However small-effect polygenes, like strong single genes, segregate at meiosis, display dominance and recessiveness and are transmitted in

216

linked blocks. Inheritance of these blocks of weak genes appears to be a major factor in the cause of many, if not most congenital anatomical malformations. The other factors are the extent to which these inherited abnormal genes are diluted by normal gene blocks and the influence of environmental agents.

Although polygenic inheritance seems a rather vague concept, its importance in congenital malformations is substantial. The incidence of all the important congenital malformations is 10 to 40 times higher in 1st degree relatives, e.g. siblings, than in the general population. Because it is polygenic (as opposed to monogenic) inheritance, the affected proportion declines sharply and progressively in 2nd and 3rd degree relatives. However, like single gene mutations, degrees of 'penetrance' (likelihood of manifestation) occur. In families where two 1st degree relatives are already affected, there is an increased chance of further cases. A similarly increased risk, over and above the 10 to 40 times risk generally present, is seen when the malformation is severe rather than mild or partial. All this data fits well with the central concept of polygenic inheritance in which there is a gradation of total liability to the disease which becomes manifest when a certain threshold is passed. The alternative explanation for this familial pattern of congenital malformation is monogenic inheritance with variable manifestation (penetrance). At present this does not fit the observed facts as regards siblings, parents and twins.

Environment is well recognised to influence the operation of polygenic inheritance, common examples being inherited resistance to tuberculosis in relation to risk of infection and inherited height in relation to nutrition. Congenital malformations are a good example of this interrelationship because a number of substances are known which can cause anatomical deformities in the newborn often of one particular part of the body. Such agents are known as teratogens and fall into three classes, viruses, irradiation or chemicals.

Irradiation, mainly X-rays, gamma rays or beta particles may act chiefly by causing faulty chromosomal separation, a subject already discussed (p. 211). Certainly the survivors of the Hiroshima atomic bomb explosion produced a high proportion of deformed babies and for this reason pregnant women are X-rayed as infrequently as possible.

Most viruses do not pass the placental barrier. The most important exception is rubella (German measles) which is liable to produce serious defects if the mother becomes infected in the early months of pregnancy. The fetus itself becomes infected and may suffer mental subnormality, cardiac malformations, blindness or deafness. In the case of deafness at least, there is good evidence that its appearance depends upon a polygenic type of inherited predisposition as outlined above. In other words even the rubella virus needs a genetically susceptible fetus, if it is to produce damage.

Cytomegalic inclusion virus is apt to cause fetal infection *in utero* by placental growth. Such infection usually leads to stillbirth but survivors may show defective cerebral development.

Chemical teratogens have aroused much interest because of the disastrous effects of thalidomide, an otherwise useful sedative. Pregnant women taking this substance produced a high proportion of children with badly deformed arms or legs. Chemical teratogens show high species specificity and thalidomide has only weak effects on the offspring of rats, mice and rabbits. Some teratogens have known destructive effects on the developing cells of the various anatomical systems of the fetus. In this category are cytotoxic drugs, e.g. cyclophosphamide, used to destroy rapidly dividing cancer cells, and also paradoxically, cancer-inducing compounds such as dimethylnitrosamine. There is a long list of chemicals which have been found to cause general or specific anatomical malformations in various species, but information relating directly to man is scanty. A variety of environmental pollutants have been suggested, e.g. arsenic, cadmium, mercury, indium and lead. Excess of vitamin A has been proposed as a cause of brain malformation, and also mouldy potatoes. Because of these uncertainties it is standard practice not to give new drugs to pregnant women.

If it is possible to summarise this complex situation it is probably true to say that the major factor in the causation of congenital anatomical malformations is polygenic inheritance. Whether this inheritance is expressed as a malformation may depend upon the presence of certain chemicals in foods, drugs or in the atmosphere. It is not yet possible to be certain which chemicals have this potential for harm. In addition, substances exist which are powerful inducers of malformations, probably even in the absence of polygenic predisposition, but these compounds are not commonly encountered. Viruses, notably rubella, may form an intermediate group in which polygenic inheritance is more important than when powerful cytotoxic or teratogenic drugs are involved. At present it is not possible easily to disentangle environmental influences operating after fertilisation from polygenic inherited susceptibility.

Bibliography *(Chapters 30, 31, 32, 33)*

British Medical Bulletin 1976 Human malformations vol 32, no 1. British Council, London

Nicholson B E (designer) Inborn errors of metabolism-chart, 12th edn. Koch-Light Ltd

Roberts J A, Pembery M E 1978 Introduction to medical genetics 7th edn. Oxford University Press, Oxford

Woollam D A, Morris G M (eds) 1974 Experimental embryology and teratology Vol I. Elek, London

Yumis J J, Chandler M E 1977 The chromosomes of man—clinical and histological significance. American Journal of Pathology 88: 466

34

The HLA system and disease

The red cell antigens which constitute the well-known blood groups are very familiar. More recently it has been discovered that most human body cells have on their surface a number of histocompatability (HLA) antigens. These surface antigens are the markers by which the cells of an individual 'recognise' the other cells from the same individual and 'accept' them while rejecting cells from other individuals. The sensitivity of this individual recognition system is due to the large number of possible antigen permutations. This is in turn due to the large number of alleles (alternative genes) in the genes coding for the surface antigens. The HLA system comprises 4 or 5 gene loci on chromosome number 6 (in mice it is chromosome 17). They are lettered A, B, C and D and DR. It is not yet clear whether D and DR are identical but they probably are. There are at least 20 different antigens coded for by the A locus, another 20 or more by the B locus, at least 5 for the C locus and at least 8 for the D locus (or DR locus). Each individual has 2 antigens from each locus. The enormous number of permutations which is the basis of immunological individuality thus becomes clear. New antigens are constantly being discovered and the letter W (e.g. DRW) is often inserted to show a provisional designation (W = workshop). The individual HLA antigens are numbered, e.g. A1, A2 etc: B5, B8; C3, D3 or DR3 or DRW3. Obviously each lettered and numbered surface antigen corresponds to a particular gene on chromosome 6. (Fig. 34.1). The eight antigens are inherited in ordinary Mendelian fashion except that there is a tendency for particular combinations to be inherited together, e.g. DR3 and B8. This partner-

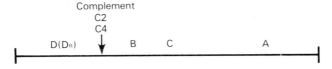

Fig. 34.1 The location of HLA genes and genes coding for complement components C2, C4 on chromosome 6 in humans.

ship is known as linkage disequilibrium, which simply means that two genes are associated more often than would be predicted by chance or random association. Linkage disequilibrium has been important in working out the disease associations of the HLA system.

It is curious that there is now no agreement as to the words for which 'HLA' stands. Human or histocompatability; lymphoid, leucocyte or locus; antigen or simply 'A' are all used. However the antigens themselves are glycoproteins of 45000 daltons attached non-covalently to β_2 microglobulins of 11600 daltons. They are virtually absent from erythrocytes, fat, brain and aorta, most easily demonstrated on lymphocytes but also present on platelets, polymorphs, monocytes, and the cells of lung, liver, intestine, kidney and heart.

Because the HLA system in mice was found to be linked to the inheritance of certain diseases, similar associations were looked for in man. Hodgkins disease and leukaemia were initially investigated but the first major association was found between HLA B27 and ankylosing spondylitis, a form of rheumatoid arthritis affecting the spine. About 90 per cent of these patients have the B27 surface antigen (and the corresponding gene). However no more than 3 per cent of individuals with the B27 antigen have overt ankylosing spondylitis, although more may have occult disease.

Another important association is with multiple sclerosis, a progressive demyelination of the central nervous system due to faulty oligodendrocyte function (p. 159). The association reported was with HLA A3, then with B7 and finally a stronger association with DR2. In other words, the real association is with DR2 and the relationship with A3 and B7 is due to linkage disequilibrium between these 3 genes, i.e. they tend to be inherited together, for reasons which are unknown.

A group of auto-immune diseases (p. 54) is associated with inheritance of the B8, D3 genetic package. These include myasthaenia gravis in which 80 per cent of the patients have B8, DR3 antigens, primary thyrotoxicosis (Graves' disease) and chronic active hepatitis. Also in the B8, DR3 group is coeliac disease (gluten enteropathy) not unequivocally auto-immune by other criteria, but with a B8, DR3 incidence of almost 90 per cent.

There is another group of diseases associated with auto-antibodies linked with the genetic package of B8, DR3 and DR4. These are Type I (juvenile onset) diabetes mellitus (p. 226) and rheumatoid arthritis.

The HLA antigen A3 is associated with the iron storage disease haemochromatosis and HLA C6 with psoriasis, a chronic skin disease. Both these conditions are of unknown aetiology and neither is seriously suspected to be auto-immune.

The mechanism whereby HLA inheritance determines disease is

unknown. What is certain is that in most cases the patient inherits not the disease itself but a susceptibility to the environmental factors which cause it. HLA inheritance thus differs from classical Mendelian inheritance where the gene itself specifies the disease but has some affinity with polygenic inheritance e.g. of congenital malformations, where environmental factors also interreact with inherited predisposition.

HLA associated disease differs from ordinary genetic disease in another important respect, in that the gene determining disease susceptibility may not be the HLA gene itself but a quite different gene which is however so close spatially to the HLA gene on chromosome 6, that the two are transmitted together in the same parcel of DNA. This means invoking the concept of linkage disequilibrium again. The idea however, is not purely hypothetical. Very close to the D or DR locus on chromosome 6 is the gene which codes for the second and fourth components of complement. We have already seen how complement deficiencies might precipitate auto-immune disease (p. 57).

Another possibility which is very much alive is that the D or DR locus might code for the vital surface recognition antigens which enable T cells, B cells and macrophages to co-operate in the production of antibodies to foreign antigens and in the non-production of antibodies to self antigens (p. 56). This appears to be the case in the mouse, where the chromosome region which corresponds to the D locus of man is the seat of the IR (immune recognition) gene. The IR antigens coded for by this gene are detectable on B cells, T cells and macrophages.

Because of their relationship to immune recognition and complement genes, it is easy to see how HLA genes and antigens, either directly or because of linkage disequilibrium, could become 'markers' of disease due to some disturbance of immuno-regulation. Such disturbances are likely to be too subtle to become manifest as obvious immuno-deficiency leading, for example to recurrent infection.

Disordered immunoregulation may be present in patients with the B8/DR3 haplotype, who eliminate hepatitis B virus more quickly than controls. Perhaps this enhances the danger of persistent occult virus infection. Similarly, patients with the B27 antigen are more likely to develop arthritis after bowel infections than non B27 controls and some invading bacteria seem to persist longer in their intestine. In such patients certain combinations of immune recognition genes could create disorder in the interplay of T cells, B cells and macrophages so that undesirable antibodies appear and desirable antibodies are lacking.

There are alternative possibilities. The HLA genes could be in linkage disequilibrium with genes directly controlling enzyme function, e.g. iron metabolism in haemochromatosis. In other cases there could be cross-reactivity between certain HLA surface antigens on the one hand and viruses or bacteria on the other. This would lead to the production of auto-antibodies when the apropriate micro-organisms were encountered.

These possibilities are all illustrated in current speculation about multiple sclerosis. The disease could be due to a gene of low penetrance in linkage disequilibrium with the DR gene (see Table 34.1) and causing lack of some enzyme essential for normal oligodendrocyte function. It seems more likely however that the DR antigen is a marker

Table 34.1 HLA associations

HLA antigen	Associations
D(R)W3 B8	Coeliac disease Chronic active hepatitis Myasthenia gravis Graves disease (thyrotoxicosis)
D(R)W3 D(R)W4 B8	Type I diabetes Rheumatoid arthritis Myasthenia gravis (Japanese)
D(R)W2 D(R)W4 D(R)6 B27	Multiple sclerosis (Europe, Canada, Australia) Multiple sclerosis (Italy) Multiple sclerosis (Japan) Ankylosing spondylitis Reiters disease
A3	Haemochromatosis
CW6	Psoriasis

for susceptibility to a virus, as in type I diabetes (p. 228). An abnormal response in childhood to a virus (e.g. measles or canine distemper) could lead to persistence of the virus in adult life leading in turn, as explained on p. 57, to an auto-immune reaction which happens to damage oligodendrocytes. The typical exacerbations and remissions of the disease could be due to recurrent re-infection by the virus, to changes in the balance of suppressor and helper T cells (p. 38) resulting in fluctuations in the auto-immune response or to non-specific factors.

It will be apparent that much of what is written above is speculation. What is certain is that the HLA system has brought genetics, virology, bacteriology, immunology and pathology into fruitful linkage disequilibrium and that a major chapter in the understanding of disease is in the process of development.

Bibliography

Bodmer W F 1980 The HLA system and disease. Journal of the Royal College of Physicians of London 14: 43

35

Gout, diabetes and heredity

Gout

Gout is a disorder of uric acid metabolism, characterised by deposition of urate crystals in the tissues, especially in the joints, and by an increase in the concentration of uric acid in tissue fluids, including the blood plasma. Clinically the disease is characterised by recurrent attacks of very painful acute arthritis, often in the big toe. The excessive amounts of circulating urates have a predeliction to precipitate in the synovium of the joints and in the surrounding connective tissue. The reason for this selectivity is not known. In any case it is only relative, because in severe, chronic untreated examples urate precipitation may be widespread in connective tissues, heart and kidney.

In a typical case of acute gouty arthritis, the urate crystals accumulate in the synovium and excite an acute inflammatory reaction due to chemical irritation. Polymorphonuclear leucocytes accumulate and phagocytose the microcrystals. This leads to a particularly explosive release of lysosomal enzymes with activation of kinins (p. 64) which probably account for much of the pain. No doubt there is also activation of complement and release of prostaglandins. As might be predicted from the activity of the polymorphs there may also be fever due to production of endogenous pyrogen (p. 101). The acute attack eventually subsides, due presumably to excretion of the offending crystals.

Although the pathogenesis of gouty arthritis is relatively clear, that of the disease itself is complicated because of the complexity of urate metabolism and excretion. Uric acid is the end product of purine catabolism and is derived from the breakdown of nucleic acids, both endogenous and from the diet. Primary gout (as opposed to secondary gout where there is an obvious reason for urate overproduction, e.g. white cell breakdown in leukaemia) is genetically determined. There are however innumerable points in the metabolic pathway where a mutant gene could interfere. In one form, there seems to be an overproduction of the substrates which form inosinic acid, a precursor of xanthine, which in turn yields uric acid. There may be increased activity of the enzymes which form inosinic acid. There may be decreased production of adenine or guanine nucleotides with loss of negative feedback control of uric acid production.

The excretion of urate also is complex, involving glomerular filtration, tubular reabsorption then tubular secretion prior to excretion. These processes too may be subject to genetically determined disorders.

One rare form of gout, inherited via an X-linked recessive gene and called the Lesch-Nyhan syndrome, does have a well worked out biochemical basis. This is lack of an enzyme, absence of which leads to increased purine synthesis because free purine bases can no longer be reconverted to their nucleotides.

What is now clear is that gout and hyperuricaemia are merely phenotypic expressions of a very wide variety of possible metabolic disturbances. As might be expected, therefore, although most cases have a familial basis the genetics are extremely complicated. Inheritance as an autosomal variant with increased chance of expression in the male is probably the commonest pattern.

Diabetes mellitus

This common condition in one form or another affects about 2 per cent of the population in general and about 1 in 10 000 children. It can be defined as an absolute or relative deficiency of insulin causing defective carbohydrate utilisation with a raised blood glucose concentration. This latter may be detected in the fasting state (over 120 mg/dl) or 2 hours after a dose of oral glucose (180 mg/dl).

The profound effects of insulin lack are thought to result mainly from the inability of glucose in the absence of insulin to enter vital body cells such as muscle or liver. As a result blood glucose rises, glucose appears in the urine and there is excessive metabolism of fat to replace the carbohydrate which is no longer available. This lipid breakdown may lead to an accumulation of keto acids which can adversely affect the brain and cause the patient to lapse into coma. In the long term, the excessive amounts of lipid components in the circulation may be a major factor in the increased speed with which diabetics develop atheroma compared with non-diabetics of comparable age (p. 135). Diabetics also suffer from non-atheromatous degeneration of arterioles and capillaries, especially in the kidney and in the retina, leading to renal failure and blindness respectively. They also have an increased risk of infection notably from tuberculosis or of the urinary tract. This deadly triad of atheroma, microangiopathy and infection accounts for the elevated mortality rate of diabetics as compared with the population as a whole. Adequate treatment has of course enormously reduced the death rate from acute complications such as ketotic coma but has had a less dramatic effect on death from long-term complications.

Diabetes may be secondary to endocrine disorders, notably of the pituitary or adrenal glands, it may be secondary to pancreatic destruction, e.g. by chronic pancreatitis or to drugs or to rare inherited syndromes. In addition there are other groups, e.g. pregnant mothers or obese subjects who develop hyperglycaemia but revert to normal when pregnancy is over and weight is reduced.

The great majority of diabetes is however primary diabetes, i.e. caused by no other recognised disease. It is known that there are two main types of diabetes, type I or insulin dependent, also known as juvenile diabetes and type II, or insulin independent also known as maturity onset diabetes. It should be explained that the term 'insulin dependent' in this context means that the diabetes is demonstrably associated with an absolute diminution in the amount of insulin in the circulation or pancreas and is relieved by administration of insulin. 'Insulin independent' means that there is usually no demonstrable absolute deficiency of insulin in the circulation although the diabetes may nevertheless respond to therapeutic administration of 'excess' of insulin.

Undoubtedly the greatest advance in separating primary diabetes into at least 2 main types has been the discovery and analysis of the HLA system of histocompatibility antigens. Their importance, as explained in the previous chapter, lies in their special relationship to genes carrying susceptibility or resistance to particular diseases.

It is now recognised that four HLA antigens have a significant positive correlation with type I diabetes. These are HLA B8, B15, B18 and B40. By contrast HLA B7 may indicate a decreased risk of diabetes. More recent analysis of the HLA system has shown that the 'B' series mentioned above are merely 'secondary' markers for diabetic susceptibility and that the 'final' HLA markers for genetic susceptibility to type I diabetes are the lymphocyte antigens DR3, (related to B8 and B18) and DR4 (related to B15 and probably B40). The 'final' antigen possibly a marker for resistance to diabetes is DR2, related to B7. It is of interest that the degree of susceptibility conferred by possession of one antigen, e.g. B8 is additive to that conferred by B15. This raises the possibility that the mechanisms of inheritance may be Mendelian autosomal recessive but there are other probably more likely explanations related to the spatial localisation of the genes on the chromosome, e.g. 'overdominance' or 'epistasis'. More important, the evidence suggests that DR3 and DR4 relate to separate disease susceptibility genes each conferring its own brand of liability to diabetes.

How then does this complicated genetic analysis help us to understand the pathology of diabetes mellitus? The most important point is that the HLA antigens discussed above are probably markers for genes determining the nature of the immune response. There is no evidence at all that genetic factors alone can account for type I diabetes but a great deal of evidence that they do so in combination with environmental factors. Of these, the one thought most likely to be involved is the coxsackie B virus. This is known to sometimes favour a pancreatic localisation although attempts to isolate it from the pancreas in humans are usually unsuccessful. The presence of DR2 and DR3 antigens correlates well with high titres of neutralising antibody to coxsackie B but not with any other virus tested. The only other viral correlation with type I diabetes so far reported is congenital rubella infection. However, type I diabetes has a seasonal variation in onset which suggests infection by more than one virus.

It seems then that part of the genetic predisposition to type I diabetes is related to a susceptibility of pancreatic islet cells to infection and destruction by coxsackie B virus. Early cases of the disease show degeneration and progressive disappearance of beta cells in the islets and infiltration of the islets with lymphocytes.

Another factor is the similar correlation which exists between DR2 and DR3 antigens and the presence of high titres of anti-islet cell auto-antibodies. High titres of antibody to autologous insulin are also often present. In other words, there is very substantial evidence of coxsackie B virus infection and of auto-immunity to islet cells and autologous insulin in patients with type I diabetes, both viral infection and auto-immunity apparently being genetically determined.

At least 80 per cent of islet cells need to be destroyed before serious insulin deficiency occurs. This means that the initial damage must occur well before the disease is apparent. Indeed, anti-islet cell antibody has often been found before diabetes is obvious. The evidence suggests that type I insulin dependent diabetes results either from cumulative islet cell destruction, e.g. by repeated exposure to virus, or continuous islet cell destruction, e.g. by auto-immunity following initial exposure to virus. In either case, it seems that an immunological abnormality exists, coded for by immune response genes in linkage disequilibrium

Type II diabetes differs from type I in that onset is not predominantly in youth (although it may start in the young); type II diabetics are not prone to ketosis, have no evidence of auto-immunity or special evidence of coxsackie virus infection. Type II diabetes has no relationship with HLA antigens and is not usually associated with low levels of insulin. Type II diabetes may or may not be associated with obesity and may or may not require insulin to control the hyperglycaemia.

Type II diabetes is essentially an inability of the body to respond appropriately and quickly to a rise in blood glucose concentration. Its pathogenesis remains obscure. It may result from a failure of insulin to respond to blood glucose changes; from an excessive proportion of protein-bound to unbound insulin in the circulation; from the presence of endogenous insulin inhibitors or from the presence of abnormal insulin which may be biologically ineffective or even antigenic. The most favoured view now, however, is that there is defective insulin receptor concentration or affinity which leads to insulin resistance by the affected target cells.

It is important to appreciate that type II diabetes, like the type I variety is to a large extent genetically determined. The difference is that type I diabetes has its basis in disease-susceptibility genes with HLA markers, whereas type II diabetes has a more familiar pattern of Mendelian inheritance, albeit variable as regards dominance, recessivity and penetrance.

Bibliography

Cudworth A G, Festenstein H 1978 HLA genetic heterogeneity in diabetes mellitus. British Medical Bulletin 34: 285

Rajan K T, Wilkins M, Barr B, Henderson B 1978 Urate deposition and inflammation. European Journal of Rheumatology and Inflammation 1: 92

Stanbury J B, Wyngaarden J B, Fredrickson D S 1978 The metabolic basis of inherited disease. 4th ed. McGraw-Hill, New York

36

Neoplasia

Neoplasia means new growth and a neoplasm (commonly known also as a tumour) is an area of tissue whose growth has outstripped and become independent of the adjoining tissue. By far the most important group of neoplasms are those known generically as cancer. Synonyms for cancer are malignant growths or malignant neoplasms. The single word 'growth' is often used as a euphemism for malignant neoplasm, an indication of the terror which the word cancer tends to inspire, often unnecessarily.

Taxonomy tends to be regarded as the dullest part of any scientific subject. In the study of neoplasia, however, taxonomy has always been crucial because the label given to a tumour by a pathologist based on its appearance under the light microscope is the most important guide to the patient's prospects of being alive 1, 5 or 15 years later.

The most basic and important taxonomic decision about a neoplasm is whether it is benign or malignant. This decision is usually the pathologist's job and is his most important task in hospital practice. A benign tumour is slow growing, well demarcated from the surrounding tissues, is composed of cells indistinguishable from those from which it is derived, does not infiltrate into adjacent tissues or spread to distant organs and does not threaten life unless it happens to interfere with some function necessary for survival. In practice a benign tumour is dangerous only if it encroaches on a vital structure like the brain or if it produces something harmful, such as an excess of a hormone (Table 36.1).

A malignant tumour has characteristics which are the opposite of benign. Cancer is typically fast growing, poorly demarcated from surrounding tissues, is composed of cells which often differ markedly from the cells of origin, infiltrates adjacent tissues and spreads to distant organs and sooner or later invariably causes death if untreated no matter where it arises.

From the patient's point of view the differentiation between malignancy and non-malignancy may be one of the most important decisions of his life. The two types of tumour are distinguished by an

Table 36.1 The main features of benign and malignant tumours

Benign	Malignant
Slow growing	Fast growing
Non-infiltrating	Infiltrating
Resembles parent tissue	Differs from parent tissue
Cells normal	Cells abnormal
Does not spread to distant sites	Spreads to distant sites
Only kills if damaging vital function	Always kills if untreated

elaborate classification, each term having a precise meaning. Ignorance or misunderstanding of this terminology by any of his medical attendants could have grave consequences for the patient. The broad classification of human tumours is given in the accompanying table (Table 36.2).

The table shows certain terms, i.e. carcinoma, epithelioma, sarcoma, lymphoma, invariably indicate a malignant tumour. Benign tumours are usually designated by the parent tissue combined with the suffix 'oma', e.g. fibroma, lipoma. It shows also that certain tissues produce only tumours considered malignant. No attempt has been made in the table to subdivide epithelial tumours systematically. More complete classifications of epithelial neoplasms are quite elaborate. In practice, attention is given both to the cell type and to the organ from

Table 36.2 Classification of tumours

Tissue of origin	Benign	Malignant
Epithelium	Adenoma	Carcinoma
	Papilloma	Epithelioma
	Naevus	
	Benign melanoma	Malignant melanoma
Mesenchyme		
(a) Connective tissue	Fibroma	Fibrosarcoma
(b) Smooth muscle	Leiomyoma	Leiomyosarcoma
(c) Striated muscle	Rhabdomyoma	Rhabdomyosarcoma
(d) Connective tissue	Myxoma	Myxosarcoma
(e) Cartilage	Chondroma	Chondrosarcoma
(f) Fat	Lipoma	Liposarcoma
(g) Bone	Osteoma	Osteosarcoma
(h) Vessels	Angioma	Angiosarcoma
(i) Lymphoid tissue	—	Lymphoma
(j) Haemopoetic tissue	—	Leukaemia
(k) Mesothelium	—	Mesothelioma
(l) Meninges	Meningioma	—
(m) CNS glial cells	—	Glioma
(n) Nerve sheath	Neurofibroma	Neurofibrosarcoma
Embryonic rests	Teratoma	Malignant teratoma

which the tumour originates, e.g. bronchogenic adenocarcinoma. This means a malignant epithelial tumour (carcinoma) derived from glandular epithelium (adeno) from the bronchus (bronchogenic). Correct use of conventional taxonomy is essential not only to distinguish between benign and malignant tumours but also to identify different sorts of malignancies, since these vary enormously in their clinical behaviour and response to treatment. To give an example not quoted in the table, a carcinoma of the testis derived from seminiferous tubules (seminoma) has a very good prognosis, a carcinoma of the testis derived from totipotential cells (embryonal carcinoma, choriocarcinoma) has a very poor prognosis. Tissue pathologists have a reputation for being obsessed with classifications and nomenclature. Their preoccupation should now be understandable.

Benign tumours

In general these are not of great clinical importance. They resemble the parent tissue closely and are surrounded either by a fibrous capsule or a zone of compressed parent tissue, so are easily removed by the surgeon, sometimes as easily as separating a pea from its pod (Fig. 36.1). Because of their slow rate of growth it is rare to see mitosis in these tumours and they may take many years to come to the patient's notice. However, since they compress surrounding tissue they presumably comprise a localised group of cells whose growth rate exceeds that of surrounding cells. The adjacent normal tissues bar the exten-

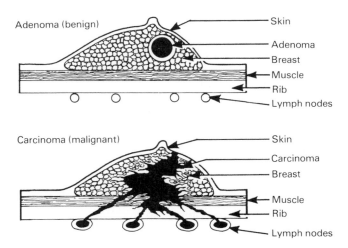

Fig. 36.1 The differences between a benign (adenoma) and a malignant (carcinoma) tumour of the breast.

sion of the tumour which then exerts pressure on them. Thus the cells of benign tumours behave abnormally in their growth pattern but normally in their failure to breach natural boundaries. The cells of benign tumours are usually normal in their capacity to form their natural products whether it be collagen of parathormone. This can be an embarrassment to homeostasis, if hormones produced by endocrine adenomas are secreted in excess of bodily requirements. In such cases surgical removal is usually necessary. The compression of surrounding structures by a benign tumour may also necessitate its removal, e.g. in the brain or spinal canal.

Perhaps the most important question both theoretically and practically about benign tumours is whether they become malignant, i.e. invade surrounding tissues, spread to distant organs and lose the features of their parent cells. Unfortunately it is a difficult question to answer simply. The great majority of benign tumours never acquire these characteristics. There are, however, instances where a carcinoma develops at the site of a tumour which was found on previous examination to have the structural features of a benign tumour. Modern opinion inclines to the view that although the original neoplasm may have had the histological features of a benign tumour, it was in fact malignant but in a pre-invasive phase. This is borne out by the fact that such transformations from benign to malignant almost always occur in specific, well-recognised situations. Three examples are the genetically determined multiple papilloma of the colon (familial polyposis), papilloma of the bladder and adenoma of the bronchus. All three are essentially malignant tumours which happen to be diagnosed before they have fully expressed their potential for loss of cell differentiation, invasiveness and spread to distant organs. In the same way a melanoma may be present for some time before becoming obviously malignant but this does not mean that naevi, e.g. pigmented moles, become cancerous. Most authorities would say that they did not do so.

The nature of the cellular change in benign neoplasia has naturally received less attention from research workers than cancer itself. A benign tumour can be regarded as a partial and incomplete manifestation of the cell transformation which occurs in malignancy. Alternatively, it can be viewed as a localised example of the cellular hyperplasia described in a previous chapter as occurring in the breast, prostate, thyroid and other organs (Ch. 29). In all probability both suggestions are true, one applying to some benign tumours and one applying to the others.

A special example of a benign tumour is the hamartoma, derived from 'rests' of embryonic origin. They can therefore be regarded as developmental anomalies rather than as true tumours. Hamartomas are found in many different organs and tissues.

Malignant tumours

How cancer becomes apparent depends on the nature of the tumour and on the site of its growth. It may present as a painless lump, e.g. in the breast, as loss of weight and general ill-health or as some specific and alarming symptom such as haematemesis (coughing up blood). Needless to say all these events also occur commonly because of trivial illness.

In spite of this variation in the clinical presentation of cancer it is possible to reconstruct some fairly typical natural histories of malignant disease. In a case of carcinoma of the stomach a middle aged or elderly man may present with loss of weight and appetite and is found to have lost 30 lbs in weight fairly rapidly. He looks pale and unwell. A tumour is found in his stomach by using special X-ray techniques and surgical removal is undertaken. However, at operation numerous small white nodules are found in the peritoneum and the mesenteric and paraortic lymph nodes are enlarged and filled with tumour. The liver also is enlarged and exhibits white nodules of tumour. The tumour has extended directly from the stomach into the pancreas behind. The patient recovers from the operation but a few months later becomes ill and confused, is readmitted to hospital and dies of pneumonia. A post-mortem examination reveals that the gastric cancer has spread throughout the liver and peritoneum, involves many lymph nodes even in the neck and has sent secondary deposits to the brain.

A different type of case history is that of a woman who discovers a lump in her breast. It is removed and found to be adenocarcinoma of the breast. The woman is well for 15 years, then unaccountably develops illness and back pain. She is found to have wide-spread secondary deposits of breast carcinoma and dies shortly after.

On a more cheerful note, a middle-aged man might present with an acute intestinal blockage and be found at operation to have a carcinoma of the large intestine which is removed. He remains symptom free and dies of old age 30 years later.

The first of these three cases is not necessarily the most frequent type or the most typical, but it is the most helpful as a prelude to understanding the pathology of malignant disease.

In the diagnosis and assessment of a malignant tumour the pathologist identifies the cells from which the tumour is derived, if possible observing the junction of normal and neoplastic cells. He then records the degree of differentiation of the tumour, i.e. the extent to which the individual cells and the structures formed from them resemble the parent tissues. If the glands, ducts, epithelial sheets, etc. are indistinguishable from normal the tumour is said to be fully differentiated. If the cells bear no resemblance to their cells of origin and no normal structures are formed, the tumour is said to be totally undifferentiated or anaplastic. There are of course all degrees of intermediate differentiation.

The first characteristic of the cancer cell is diminished ability to form appropriate structures such as glandular acini (Fig. 36.2). Benign tumours form such structures normally. In addition, cancer cells themselves are abnormal in a number of ways. The ratio of nucleus to cytoplasm is usually raised and the nucleus may have increased amounts of deeply staining chromatin. There may be great variation in size and shape between the cells of a malignant tumour and bizarre forms may be present, e.g. irregular multinucleate giant cells or very large hyperdiploid single nuclei whose chromosomes are increased in number and show structural abnormalities. Thus the second characteristic of malignancy is cytological aberration.

Further examination of a malignant tumour reveals that not only have the cells lost their proper orientation to each other but that they are invading adjacent tissues. A carcinoma of the intestine for example will often infiltrate the underlying submucosa and muscle coats and even the peritoneal surface. Invasion of veins and lymphatic vessels is

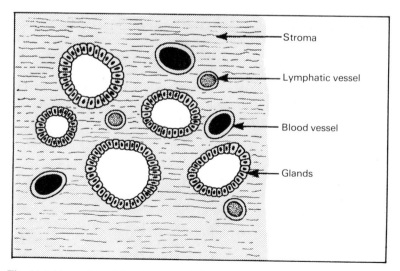

Fig. 36.2 Normal glandular tissue, e.g. in breast or large intestine showing normal architecture of epithelial glands and related structures.

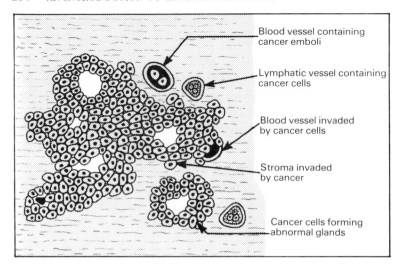

Blood vessel containing cancer emboli

Lymphatic vessel containing cancer cells

Blood vessel invaded by cancer cells

Stroma invaded by cancer

Cancer cells forming abnormal glands

Fig. 36.3 Cancerous glandular tissue involving adjacent tissues, lymphatics and blood vessels. Note loss of normal glandular arrangement.

common. Thus the third and diagnostically the most important characteristic of malignancy is infiltration and invasion (Fig. 36.3).

Mitotic figures may be seen in large numbers, indicating a high rate of growth. Malignant tumours induce the formation of new blood vessels which keep them supplied with nutriment and this may be a limiting factor in their growth. If the tumour outstrips its blood supply its centre will become ischaemic and necrotic. Leucocytic exudation of lymphocytes, macrophages and granulocytes is also sometimes apparent.

In some cases a malignant tumour is seen not to have broken through its basement membrane nor to have penetrated beyond the cell layer from which it originated. This is known as *carcinoma-in-situ* and may take many years to become fully invasive, so that resection at this stage will usually result in cure.

Malignant tumours may spead to adjacent organs and tissues by direct extension and invasion; to draining lymph nodes by way of embolisation or permeation of lymphatic channels; into body cavities by shedding free cancer cells or to distant organs by way of the blood stream following penetration of veins. All such extensions of the tumour beyond its primary site of origin are known as metastasis or secondary growth and in general carry a poor prognosis. Indeed, reference to the hypothetical case histories related above (p. 234), will make it obvious that the occurrence or non-occurrence of metastasis is a major factor in determining the curability of a particular instance of malignant disease.

In general, three factors determine the likelihood of secondary spread. These are the nature of the tumour itself, the resistance of the host and the susceptibility of the organ to which the tumour spreads. To take these in order, sarcomas, i.e. malignant tumours of connective tissue, tend to spread early by the blood stream because they grow rapidly, invade veins and the sarcoma cells have low adhesiveness to each other. On the other hand, certain carcinomas of skin epithelium never spread by the blood stream and reach local lymph nodes only after they have caused immense local destruction, usually of the face, where such tumours (basal cell carcinomas) most frequently occur. Of course, nowadays these cancers are dealt with before they reach an advanced stage and because they spread so reluctantly, are in fact easier to cure than simple plantar warts.

Host resistance is of enormous importance in determining metastasis and the subject is essentially that of cancer immunology which is dealt with later (p. 267). The body's chances of rejecting tumour cells is greater if the main tumour mass is removed. If this is achieved and secondary deposits nevertheless appear, it would seem that a failure of the immune mechanism has occurred. This seems to happen particularly in cancer of the breast, where widespread metastasis may develop many years after apparent cure of the primary tumour by surgical removal. Of course if secondary deposits have had time to become established before the primary cancer is excised, the immunological mechanism has little chance of overcoming them.

The soil in which the wandering cancer cell lodges also plays a large part in determining whether a secondary deposit develops. Every malignant tumour probably discharges showers of malignant cells into the lymph and blood but only a small proportion of these potential seedlings manage to take hold and grow. As we have seen, immunological factors probably play a large part in determining this outcome. However, some organs, e.g. spleen, or skeletal muscle only rarely allow secondary tumours to develop whereas others, e.g. bones, liver and brain are common sites of metastasis. No satisfactory explanation of these differences is available, although many hypotheses have been advanced, based on the anatomical and functional peculiarities of the organs and tissues concerned.

Bibliography

Willis R A 1973 Pathology of tumours, 5th edn. Butterworth, London

37

The properties of cancer cells

It would be surprising even to the most cynical, if the vast effort devoted to cancer research in the laboratory has not yielded some information which would help in our understanding of the behaviour of cancer in man. Many techniques have been used to this end of which cell culture has been the most profitable.

In cell or tissue culture cells are kept in artificial media in incubators. Under these conditions the abnormally rapid growth of malignant tumours is matched by speedy proliferation of cancer cells compared with their normal counterparts. Cancer cells cultured in this way can be from a malignant tumour that has arisen spontaneously or can be cells separated from a similar tumour induced experimentally in an animal by giving it a cancer-inducing virus (p. 246) or a carcinogenic chemical (p. 252). Another way of obtaining cancer cells for study outside the body is to obtain normal cells in tissue culture and then to make them malignant by treating them with the viruses or chemicals just mentioned. Cultures derived from any one of these three sources are described as transformed, although the term is most commonly used in relation to cells converted to malignant behaviour during *in vitro* cultivation.

Transformed cells not only increase rapidly in number but show the abnormal karyotypes (chromosome patterns) observed in the natural tumours. Cancer cells in culture will continue dividing until the mass reaches a critical size and ceases to grow. This brake is due to lack of nutrition of the innermost cells, for if the culture is transferred to a living animal as host and acquires its own blood supply by stimulating growth of new vessels, it will grow until the host is killed.

The loss of differentiation seen in malignant tumours has its counterpart in the progressive disappearance of parental tissue characteristics found when cancer cells are cultured *in vitro*. This is apparent as characteristic features of cell size, shape and arrangement cease to be demonstrable. The electron microscope usually reveals a progressive simplification of cell structure and changes in distribution of nuclear chromatin. Biochemically, metabolic differences may be observed, e.g. cancer cells tend to be much more dependent on glycolysis than their normal counterparts which rely on aerobic respiration. However, it is important to appreciate that differences of this sort are more likely to be a result of the malignant change than its cause.

Occasionally, loss of differentiation can be shown to be accompanied by disappearance of a particular specialised biochemical function. In primary carcinoma of the liver the malignant liver cells lose the ability to respond to the feedback mechanism which normally regulates the blood cholestrol level. However, a de-differentiated cell is just as likely to acquire functions as to lose them. Thus cultured explants of bronchial carcinoma as well as the cancer growing *in vivo* may synthesise and secrete peptide hormones such as ACTH or parathormone, substances which are certainly not formed by non-cancerous bronchial epithelium. None of these peculiarities give much of a clue as to the cause or mechanism of cancer, but they corroborate the structural evidence indicating loss by the cancer cell of its status as a unit in an organ of defined and limited capabilities.

Although these changes are important, the essential criterion of whether or not a cell has suffered malignant transformation is its ability to survive and grow when transplanted to another living host. Even in the absence of immune rejection (p. 51) non-transformed, i.e. non-cancerous adult cells will not normally grow when transplanted to another animal. Indeed, most normal adult cell lines grow with difficulty when transplanted to tissue culture *in vitro* under ideal conditions. Cancer cells are much more likely to proliferate in either or both situations and can be seen therefore to have a remarkable capacity for independent survival and multiplication. The direct result of their successful growth after transplantation to another animal is death of the host. This is the ultimate proof that malignant transformation of the inoculated cells had taken place.

The cultivation outside the body of transformed cells, whether obtained artificially or from pre-existing tumours, has provided an excellent opportunity to identify the precise differences which distinguish a malignant cell from its normal counterpart.

The first point to emerge is that the essential change occurs in the transformed cell itself and that malignancy is not merely the removal of competing normal cells so that a few hardy survivors can overgrow the rest. This has been shown very directly by transforming a single cultured cell with a cancer-inducing chemical, then allowing the transformed cell to divide and observing that all of its progeny retained their malignant characteristics in spite of the fact that the transforming chemical was no longer present. This experiment was necessary because many agents (carcinogens) which induce cancer also kill cells, although there is usually little correlation between the two properties. Allowing a single cell to divide and collecting its daughter cells is known as cloning. Study of transformed cells in culture has shown that the properties of malignancy are passed from one generation to the next so that the tumour is self-perpetuating even when the stimulus is removed. This means that cancer involves a change in the genetic apparatus of the affected cells such that not only the cell itself is transformed but that all its progeny are malignant although they may differ amongst themselves in karyotype, phenotype or antigenic structure. Transformation of this sort could be due either to replacement of DNA. e.g. by viral DNA inserted into the cell after infection (p. 246), to DNA damage, e.g. by a chemical (p. 255) or to interference with a gene repressor, i.e. a protein in the cytoplasm which in a normal cell prevents certain genes from expressing their potential for malignant behaviour.

If malignant transformation were always irreversible there would be no reason to doubt that irreversible mutation in somatic cell DNA was the underlying mechanism. However, reversion of transformed cells to normal does occur and may be dramatic, as with the brain tumour grown in its malignant form in culture for thousands of cell generations and then by treatment with cyclic AMP induced to behave like an untransformed cell in culture, to differentiate specialised neural structures, to cease to cause tumours on implantation and to transmit these normal characteristics to its offspring. Similarly, primitive leukaemia cells in culture have been induced to revert to normal differentiation by treatment with certain maturation factors. Reversal of malignancy was not dependent on DNA synthesis and was undoubtedly a cytoplasmic event occurring at the level of translation rather than transcription. Reversion could have been due merely to cyclic AMP interfering with the growth pattern provoked by transformation. Alternatively, reversibility may mean that the transcriptional error that causes transformation may need to take place continuously in every cell generation of a growing tumour over long periods of time. It also shows that the genetic basis for normal differentiation may persist in cancer cells and may indeed have merely been switched off by epigenetic mechanisms. There is also the converse implication that the genetic basis for malignancy may persist in phenotypically normal cells. This could explain the phenomenon of dormancy, in which cancer recurs many years after its apparent cure.

A common sense attitude to reversibility of malignant transformation is that in some tumours malignancy may require irreversible alteration in the genes whereas in others it is sufficient merely to modify phenotypic expression of the genome leaving the DNA itself intact. It is appropriate at this point to mention experiments in which malignant cells were fused into one cytoplasm with normal cells and the resultant hybrid cells lost all malignant characteristics. This could mean that transformed genomes were overrruled by dominant genes from the normal cell, or that lost repressor molecules were donated by the normal cytoplasm allowing malignant genes to be suppressed once more, or that transformed genes were selectively lost from the hybrid. Whatever the explanation, the implication of this and of other experiments indicating the reversibility of malignancy is a hopeful one.

Reversible or not, it would seem that cancer is the result of direct or indirect interference with the genetic apparatus of the cell leading to alterations in the coding instructions which the cell receives from its DNA, leading in turn to altered structure and function. The essential nature of these alterations appears to be a lack of responsiveness to control mechanisms which regulate the behaviour of the normal cell. This lack of control affects cell movement, replication and differentiation and can be related to alterations at the surface of the transformed cell.

One of the most obvious effects of cell surface change is loss of contact inhibition of movement. When normal cells in tissue culture become confluent, movement ceases, but when the surface of a layer of transformed cells meets that of normal cells no inhibition of movement occurs and the transformed cells move over and under the others to form disorderly, multi-layered heaps. This peculiarity may be the cellular basis of malignant infiltration *in vivo*.

Another obvious effect of surface change is loss of density-dependent growth inhibition. Normal cells in culture cease to divide when a certain cell density per unit area is reached, but transformed cells fail to recognise this threshold and continue to proliferate in spite of increasing cell crowding. The phenomenon is separate from contact inhibition of movement but correlates well in general with the ability of the cells to induce tumours when implanted into living animals. The importance of the cell surface in its development is shown by the ability of treatment with proteolytic enzymes (which simply remove surface proteins) to induce normal cells to show loss of density-dependent growth inhibition.

Loss of density-dependent growth inhibition is important in explaining malignancy *in vivo* because most solid tumours do not show abnormally rapid rates of cell growth. Although in tissue culture transfomed cells often have a shorter-than-normal cell cycle time, the cell cycle times of most solid tumours *in vivo* is considerably longer than that of normal tissues, e.g. intestinal epithelial cells in a comparable state of continuous replication. In such tumours the S-phase of the mitotic cycle, i.e. the period in which the chromosomal material doubles, is prolonged and therefore is slower than in normal proliferating cells, while the proportion of cells replicating at any one time is usually lower than in normal intestinal epithelium. Thus malignancy cannot be attributed merely to rapid growth but rather to failure to respond to signals invoked by the proximity of other cells which should cause cell division to cease and permit the dividing cell to develop into a mature, non-proliferating derivative.

There are four other features of the transformed cell which show that it is essentially the result of loss of growth control. The most important is its ability to grow in the absence of a solid surface (anchorage independence). This is shown by the ease with which such cells proliferate in liquid agar cultures. Other characteristics are the rounded shape of the transformed cells in culture, the disorganisation of the cytoplasmic network of contractile fibres and the increased fluidity of the cell membrane. All these are seen in normal cells only when they are dividing.

It is apparent that the transformed cell is distinguished by its autonomy, an independence that it passes on to its descendents (Table 37.1). This autonomy may find positive as well as negative expression. Thus malignant cells from adrenal or liver in culture may continue to secrete hormones or plasma proteins whereas normal cells from these organs are unable to do so. This is part of a general loss of dependence

Table 37.1 The properties *in vitro* of normal liver cells, liver cells transformed *in vitro* and liver cells from a malignant hepatoma

	Normal	Transformed	Hepatoma
Morphology	Epithelial	Modified epithelial	Modified epithelial
Cell generation time	28 hrs	16 hrs	18 hrs
Karotype	Diploid	Aneuploid (variable)	Aneuploid
Serum protein synthesis	Yes	Yes	Yes
Contact inhibition of movement*	Yes	No	No
Density dependent growth inhibition*	Yes	No	No
Growth in suspension*	No	Yes	Yes
Agglutination by concanavalin A †	No	Yes	Yes
Tumourigenicity	No	Yes	Yes

*Indicate loss of growth control.
† Indicate changes at cell surface.

on trophic factors. Such independence is variable, so that some cultures of epithelial cancers require for their growth proximity of connective tissue (as do the corresponding normal epithelium) whereas other transformed cultures actually themselves secrete the mesenchymal trophic factors. Dependence on the proximity of dermis may explain why invasive basal cell carcinoma of the skin does not spread to distant sites. Lack of response to normal hormonal control can again be related to changes at the cell surface and may be particularly important when cancer develops in organs such as the breast, whose growth is normally tightly controlled by hormones.

The other feature of transformed cells is loss of differentiation which means, as we have already learned, disappearance of the anatomical peculiarities of that cell line. Loss of differentiation and uncontrolled proliferation are phenomena which develop independently. Although interference with differentiation in some cultures often provokes cell proliferation, arrest of proliferation does not usually by itself induce the cultures to differentiate. Cells which are already fully differentiated, e.g. keratinised squamous epithelium cannot undergo malignant transformation. To be susceptible to transformation a cell must belong to the stem cell population of the organ from which it is derived. Such cells have the capacity both to divide and to differentiate, as opposed to the fully differentiated cells which have lost the capacity to divide. In stratified epithelium the two populations are easily distinguished but in liver there is no obvious difference. In other organs which lack the power of cell replication, e.g. adult nervous tissue, stem cells are few or absent. Transformation of a stem cell *in vivo* or *in vitro* means that it is diverted from the path of differentiation to that of continued proliferation as occured during embryogenesis. The persistence of stem cells into adult life is of course essential for homeostasis in situations such as regeneration of epithelium. The ability of these stem cells to become autonomous and cause cancer is a further example of the way disease develops from perversion of a survival mechanism. In this instance since most cancers develop after the reproductive stage of life there is a clear survival advantage for the species in selecting for regenerative powers at the expense of cancer developing in later life.

The changes in the surface membranes of transformed cells which are probably responsible for their lack of response to control are fairly well documented and an active area of research. There is alteration of the receptors governing adenyl cyclase activity and a fall in cyclic AMP. Transport mechanisms at the surface are increased and there are decreased levels of glycoprotein, sialic acid and glycosyl transferase. These biochemical changes are those observed in normal cells exposed *in vitro* to growth factors such as insulin or certain serum fractions. The malignant cell could be said to behave as if it were permanently exposed to such factors even when they are not present.

The membrane changes in transformed cells are reflected in alterations of the surface antigens. These histocompatibility antigens are normally present and may be species, individual or tissue specific. Transformation is accompanied by the appearance of new cancer-associated antigens both at the cell surface (tumour rejection or surface antigens) and within the cell (T-antigens). If the transformation is induced by a virus the antigens will tend to be the same for all tumour cell lines induced by that virus even in different species. If transformation is induced by chemicals there will be a great multiplicity of cancer-associated antigens at the cell surface which will not cross-react with other tumours induced by the same chemical even when all are present in the same animal. In human cancer, malignant melanomas from different patients have been found to have tumour specific antigens in common and several types of soft tissue sarcoma have yielded cross-reacting tumour-associated surface antigens.

Another type of tumour-associated antigen found in spontaneously and experimentally transformed cells is that which occurs also in normal fetal cells but not in those of the adult. One such is the carcinoembryonic antigen (CEA) associated particularly with cancer of the colon and another is alpha-feto-protein associated with cancer of the liver. The appearance of these embryonic products is further evidence of the stem cell origin of cancer. The elaboration by malignant cells of these three types of abnormal antigen, i.e. tumour rejection (surface) antigens, T-antigens and fetal products presumably reflects the general disturbance of transcription and translation. Whether the replacement of normal cell surface antigens by tumour antigens is important in allowing cells to escape from growth control remains to be seen.

In summary, cancer occurs because stem cells in the affected organ lose their responsiveness to growth control and continue to divide so that they produce more dividing cells instead of non-proliferating, fully-differentiated progeny. Their acquisition of autonomous growth is associated with loss of specialised development and loss of the ability to stop dividing and migrating when normal cells are encountered. These changes in behaviour are associated with altered composition of the cell surface.

Bibliography

Augsberg A, Nelly 1974 In: Ioachim H L (ed) Pathobiology annual. Appleton Century Crofts, New York

Cairns J 1978 Cancer, science and society. Freeman, San Francisco

di Paulo J A, Heidelberger C 1974 In: Ts'o P.O.P and di Paulo J A (eds) Chemical carcinogenesis, part B. Dekker, New York

Post J, Hoffman H 1972 In: Ioachim H L (ed) Pathobiology annual. Appleton Century Crofts, New York

38

Viruses and cancer

In man, the only known causes of spontaneous cancer are chemicals and radiation. Viruses have not yet been proved to cause cancer in humans. Ironically, the only known cause of spontaneous cancer in animals is virus infection although chemicals and radiation as well as viruses will initiate malignant tumours when applied under experimental conditions. In animals, viruses which can cause cancer can be transmitted 'horizontally' from animal to animal, like other infections. They can also be transmitted 'vertically' from parent to child either as part of the germ cell genome (p. 248) or as an infectious agent, e.g. in the mother's milk.

At present, intense research activity is directed towards seeking evidence that viruses are a cause of cancer in man, partly because of the paradox outlined above. The only tumour-producing (oncogenic) virus in man is the papilloma virus that causes the humble wart, which is of course at most a small benign tumour. Virus (Epstein-Barr or E.B. virus) is regularly recovered from cells of one human cancer of B lymphocytes, the Burkitt lymphoma, when they are grown in culture. This tumour has a striking geographical localisation of East Africa, suggesting an infectious agent and its discovery was one of the factors leading to the present activity in oncogenic viruses. However the virus is widely distributed in the human population all over the world so it could be present in the Burkitt lymphoma mainly as a passenger. An attractive theory proposed by Burkitt himself is that the co-existence of malaria (the lymphoma and malarial regions run together) allows the E.B. virus to cause tumours by interfering with immunity (p. 34). There is also a firm association (not necessarily cause and effect) between nasopharyngeal carcinoma and E.B. virus. This tumour occurs mostly in China and S.E. Asia and the viral genome is found in the cancer cells which lie in close association with B lymphocytes. A suggestive but less definite association exist between carcinoma of the uterine cervix and herpes simplex II virus. Favoured candidates without much supporting evidence are leukaemias, lymphomas and

Table 38.1 Oncogenic viruses

	Natural host
DNA viruses	
Adenoviruses	
Types 12, 18 and others	Man*
Papovaviruses	
Polyoma	Mouse*
SV40	Rhesus monkey*
Human papilloma	Man
Herpesviruses	
H. saimiri	Squirrel monkey*
H. ateles	Spider monkey*
Lucke virus	Frog
Marek's disease virus	Chicken
Poxviruses	
Yaba virus	Rhesus monkey
RNA viruses	
Leukoviruses	
'Leukosis' viruses	Mice, birds and cats
Bittner agent	Mouse

*These viruses are not oncogenic in their natural host.

carcinoma of the breast. For the rest, the association of viruses with human cancer is conjectural.

As pointed out earlier (p. 5) there are two types of virus depending on whether the viral core is composed of DNA or RNA. Both types cause tumours in animals but whereas all varieties of DNA virus have oncogenic potential, only one group of RNA viruses, the leukoviruses, has the ability to cause tumours (Table 38.1). This is because of the RNA viruses only the leukoviruses have an enzyme, reverse transcriptase (RNA-directed DNA polymerase), which can persuade the cell to make a DNA copy of the viral RNA. The importance of this will emerge shortly.

In some species, e.g. frog and chicken, DNA virus can be recovered from a spontaneously-arising tumour, injected into another member of the same species and a tumour will result. Two types of herpes virus behave in this way. In other species, e.g. mouse, man or monkey, DNA virus can be recovered from cells usually after growth in culture and are found to induce tumours in hosts of different species or to transform cultured cells derived from species other than that to which the host belonged. In this category come certain types of adenovirus, the SV40 and polyoma virus (which belong to the same family— papovavirus—as the human papilloma or wart virus) and other varieties of herpes virus. By contrast, the RNA leukoviruses cause cancer in the species they normally inhabit. One of these is the mouse mammary tumour virus which transmitted in the mother's milk to suckling mice causes breast cancer when the recipients grow to adulthood. The other major group is the leukosis viruses which cause spontaneous leukaemia and lymphoma in mice, birds and cats.

The best way to understand how viruses may cause cancer is to return to a suggestion made earlier in this book that many pathological situations which seem absurd, suicidal or merely incomprehensible, make sense if studied from the view point of an infecting micro-organism with a well developed survival mechanism evolved through natural selection. If a virus destroyed every cell it entered it would soon cease to exist, since virus can propagate only within living cells. As a result most viruses have differing relationships with different cells easily demonstrated in tissue culture. If the cells are destroyed by the virus they are said to be permissive, if not destroyed, non-permissive. Some viruses have the ability to multiply in certain cells without killing the cell, at least for some time. Others can propagate by a process of budding at the cell surface. There is a clear survival advantage in mutant viruses which produce mild disease and are thereby allowed to persist. The extreme example of this is the persistence of the virus in all cells of the body so that it is passed on through the ova and sperm to the next generation. This occurs with some mouse mammary tumour viruses and like its secretion in the mother's milk is a mechanism of vertical transmission. Apart from these mechanisms, however, there would be a clear survival advantage to a virus it if were able to induce its host cell itself to divide so that each daughter cell became a vehicle for a new generation of virus. We have already seen that many viruses transform cells, that transformed cells behave like cancer cells, and most important from the virus's point of view, that the essence of transformation is uncontrolled cell division.

An oncogenic virus then has the property of causing cell multiplication. It does this by converting the cell to an autonomous unit. As part of the transformation the receptors on the cell surface react as if the cell were under permanent stimulation by growth factors. This leads not only to uncontrolled proliferation, but also to the other features of malignant transformation (p. 242).

To achieve transformation, a virus has first to enter a cell and then to use its own or the cell's transcriptional apparatus (p. 15) to make a protein which directly or indirectly brings about the changes described above (p. 242). A virus possesses many genes but transformation appears to be due to only one of them, since mutant viruses exist in which this particular transforming gene is temperature sensitive, and so can be switched on or off at the experimenter's will and disassociated from the other viral genes. If the parcel of genes which the virus introduces to the cell are preponderantly cell killing (cyto-toxic) and express their potential, then there will be no opportunity for transformation because the cell will die. The transformation gene's essential property is to cause de-repression of cellular DNA synthesis and it owes this ability to the general ability of the viruses, developed through evolution, to override cellular genes.

The survival of virus in permissive cells can be achieved in several ways. The herpes group (e.g. E.B. virus) appear to persist like bacterial plasmids i.e. without integration into cellular DNA but seldom expressing all their genes, so that the cell is not destroyed.

In other cases transformation is accompanied by integration of viral DNA into cellular DNA, molecules of viral DNA fitting into different areas of the cell DNA like individual bricks in a wall. As long as it remains integrated, the viral DNA is known as provirus and cannot replicate to form new virus. The act of integration sometimes depends upon a single viral gene separate from the transformation gene. A cell which contains virus in this integrated non-infective provirus form, can be regarded as a non-permissive infected cell. Integration is reversible, however, and for infective virus to be replicated, the viral DNA must separate from the cellular DNA. Replication can be achieved by treating infected non-permissive cells with certain chemicals or by fusing them with permissive cells. The integration of oncogenic virus in a non-infective form is of great importance because it explains how a cell could be transformed by a virus and contain the virus yet the virus be undetectable by the ordinary tests used to demonstrate infective microorganisms. There is also an obvious survival value for the virus in being able to become an integral part of the host cell.

Whether or not the viral genome integrated into the cell nucleus proceeds to transcribe for viral replication depends upon the availabil-ity of suitable transcription factors in the cell and on the precise site of viral integration, since it might be located in an area of the cell genome not normally transcribed, e.g. in hetrochromatin, the dense material at the periphery of many cell nuclei. All these observations help to explain the failure to find *infective virus* in transformed cells although *viral DNA* may be demonstrable.

Most of these observations apply to the smaller oncogenic viruses such as SV40 or polyoma. Large oncogenic viruses such as adenovi-ruses or herpes virus have bigger, linear DNA genomes with more genes which may prevent survival of infected cells. Transformation may therefore be visible only when the other (lethal) genes are not expressed. As we saw above the genome of some of these larger viruses may exist in the cell in non-integrated form and still be capable of achieving cell transformation and also its own replication.

The oncogenic RNA viruses, unlike DNA viruses, can multiply inside cells without killing them, so that transformation and viral replication can occur inside the same cell. However, transformation is again independent of viral replication and occurs in permissive as well as non-permissive cells. Like DNA viruses, transformation by RNA viruses is due to a single transforming gene and oncogenic RNA viruses persuade the cell to make a DNA provirus integrated into the cell chromosomes which again may or may not be expressed, i.e. replicated and if not expressed, can be induced to do so by chemical treatment. The important point is that both DNA and RNA oncogenic viruses can persist in lines of dividing cells as a DNA provirus even if viral multiplication is absent. Some RNA leukoviruses (sarcomogenic) transform all cells they infect. Others integrate but cannot transform unaided. It is possible that the latter may become oncogenic by acquiring from a helper (e.g. sarcomogenic) virus the piece of DNA which carries the transforming gene.

To re-apply this information to the living animal it seems likely that herpes viruses cause cancer, e.g. Marek's disease of fowls or possibly Burkitt lymphoma in man, when they infect non-permissive cells in which the cell killing and viral replicating genes cannot be expressed. Cells which are permissive for Marek's disease virus do not become transformed but are instead killed.

Several hypotheses have been developed to relate these intimate relationships between cells and viruses to the possibility that viruses cause cancer in man. The best known is perhaps the oncogene hypothesis which suggests that viral genomes become incorporated in cell genomes in course of evolution and are transmitted in a repressed state from one generation to the next via the chromosomes. If these viral oncogenes become activated the cells which contain them become transformed and cancer develops. It is true that RNA leukoviruses are undoubtedly transmitted in this way but unfortunately for the hypothesis even when activated are only weakly carcinogenic.

Dulbecco's hypothesis suggests that a cellular gene regulating cell surface behaviour became part of a viral DNA genome in the course of evolution. The hybrid gene then evolved into a transforming gene with great survival value for the virus, so that virus containing it would be selected for. If the virus then infected a cell and the viral genome was expressed, it would transform the cell. If it were integrated into the cell chromosomes but not expressed, it would be available for activation to a transforming gene, e.g. by combination with an infecting sarcomogenic virus or even with another part of the cellular DNA.

Why should birds and mammals have evolved such stratagems?

Temin's protovirus hypothesis suggests that development of multicellular creatures depends on mobile packets of genes passing from one cell to another. To survive the journey the package would need to evolve a protein or lipid coat (capsid). It might also need an enzyme to transcribe DNA to RNA and back again (reverse transcriptase). In other words the mobile genetic package would be a virus. Some viruses can therefore be regarded as having evolved from the genes of higher organisms. Others probably evolved from bacteria.

The hypothesis proposes that RNA tumour viruses are a minor aberration in a normal developmental process of animals, their ability to provoke tumours being regarded as an accident. Cairns has gone further and suggested that some particularly potent tumour viruses are laboratory artifacts, in that repeated experimental infection and recovery has led to the selective breeding of strains which can cross species barriers. There is good evidence for this but it does not mean that viruses do not cause cancer outside the laboratory.

We know from warts produced in humans by papilloma viruses that viruses can cause epithelial cells to proliferate. Nevertheless, as yet the spontaneous malignant tumours of man and other mammals in which viruses are implicated appear to be either multifactorial (e.g. mammary cancer in mice) or a proliferation of cells of the lympho-medullary system associated with abnormal immune responses (e.g. Burkitt lymphoma). The major importance of research into viruses and cancer may therefore prove to be the light it sheds on the genetic initiation of malignancy within the cancer cell rather than the more obvious goal of establishing that particular viruses cause particular tumours.

Bibliography

Augsberg A Nelly 1974 In: Joachim H L (ed) Pathobiology annual. Appleton Century Crofts, New York

Cairns J 1978 In: Doll R, Vodopija L (eds) Host environment interactions in the aetiology of cancer in man. IARC, Lyon
the aetiology of cancer in man. IARC, Lyon

39

Chemicals and cancer

Although the importance of viruses is still in doubt at least some chemicals are known definitely to cause malignant tumours in man. Chemical carcinogens take a long time to produce their effect and it required Percivall Pott, an observer of genius, to discover the connection between chemicals and cancer almost 200 years ago. His observation that soot lodged in the scrotal skin in boyhood caused scrotal cancer in adult chimneysweeps initiated not only systematic cancer research but also industrial and environmental medicine, and led to the discovery of the most important group of cancer-causing chemicals. After Pott's discovery, other occupations and other soots, tars and oils were found to have similar effects, as were aromatic amines used as dyes, chromium and asbestos. The close correlation between cigarette smoking and lung cancer is almost certainly due to a chemical carcinogen or carcinogens in the inhaled tar.

As regards the number of chemicals which induce tumours in man it could be said that many are suspected but few are proven. The proven carcinogens are sufficiently small in numbers to be listed. (1) Aromatic amines, e.g. 2-napthylamine, benzidine, chlornaphazine; (2) pitches, oils and tars containing polycyclic hydrocarbons; (3) asbestos; (4) iron ore, chromium and nickel; (5) thorotrast; (6) diethylstilboestrol.

On the other hand, the number of chemicals shown to be carcinogenic in animals and therefore potentially carcinogenic for man, is very great and increasing almost daily. Some of these chemicals occur naturally, such as aflatoxin from mouldy peanuts, but most are synthetic. All chemical carcinogens require a latent period to elapse between their administration and the development of the tumour, although this varies with the chemical and with the dose. If the substance, for example a polycyclic hydrocarbon, is painted on the skin, its action is accelerated if an irritant, notably croton oil, not itself carcinogenic (a 'promoter') is applied later. As regards natural cancers it requires 10 – 40 years of exposure before the tumour becomes clinically apparent. This is well seen both in cigarette smokers (carcinoma of the bronchus) and in the aniline dye industry (carcinoma of the bladder).

Some carcinogens are effective if given by mouth, others by injection. The testing of foodstuffs, food additives, environmental pollutants etc. for cancer inducing effect, is a difficult and expensive process. As will be explained later the induction of mutation in bacteria is a useful screening test for carcinogenicity. Certainty only prevails however, when ignorance allows the experiment to be performed unwittingly in man, as in the induction of bronchogenic carcinoma by cigarettes. Working from animal experiments, one has to consider the potency of the carcinogenic substance, the type of tumours it produces and how it has to be given to do so, the type and number of species in which tumours can be provoked, and the importance of the substance for man. The sweetening agents saccharine and cyclamates may or may not be carcinogenic for man but their use certainly helps to reduce obesity which has an unquestioned mortality and morbidity.

A glance at any list of chemical carcinogens reveals a great diversity of chemical structure. This suggests either that many types of molecules may transform cells or that different carcinogens are converted in the body to a common active product. In fact as we will see later most carcinogens need to be acted on by bodily enzymes before they are effective cancer-producing agents. The final active product is known as the ultimate carcinogen and its intermediary precursor as the proximate carcinogen. All the available evidence suggests that there are many different ultimate carcinogens, indeed, almost as many as there are carcinogens themselves.

At first sight it seems strange that chemicals which are ingested as active carcinogens are much less important than those taken in as inactive precursors. However, because they are very reactive, the former interact with the lining epithelium of the respiratory and alimentary tracts which are constantly shed and discarded, taking the carcinogen with them. The precursors do not bind to and react with these lining cells and so are innocently absorbed.

We are faced therefore with a situation in which chemicals, by themselves harmless are converted by the body's own enzymes to cancer-provoking agents. The enzymes in question are the microsomal hydroxylases, the same catalysts which play a role in some liver diseases (p. 158). These drug metabolising enzymes undoubtedly evolved as a method of detoxifying harmful substances ingested or manufactured by the body. They are unusual in that their level can be greatly increased by feeding them certain substrates, i.e. they are 'inducible' enzymes.

The process of detoxication involves oxidation, hydrolysis and conjugation. Unfortunately the oxidation and hydrolysis which neutralise some poisons cause some otherwise harmless substances to form highly reactive intermediates which are cancer-producing. It might be argued that activity in these enzymes should be selected against in evolution since they cause cancer. However, undetoxified poisons would be likely to kill children or young adults of reproductive age whereas cancer is a disease of middle and old age, affecting those who have already reproduced the species. Survival advantage lies therefore with retention of the enzymes.

The polycyclic hydrocarbons are found in soot and cigarette smoke and are the most important potential carcinogens for man. They are converted to metabolic derivatives called epoxides by the microsomal hydroxylases, the epoxides being the ultimate carcinogen (Figs. 39.1 & 39.2). Aromatic amines, e.g. 2-naphthylamine and azo compounds, e.g. dimethyl amino-azobenzene also are converted to the active carcinogenic form by microsomal hydroxylases. In the case of 2-naphthylamine the active product is the N-hydroxy derivative which is then esterified by sulphate to form the ultimate carcinogen. This conversion process occurs particularly well in the bladder wall and probably accounts for the development of bladder cancer after a prolonged inadvertent intake of certain industrial dye-stuffs. Of the compounds containing nitrosogroups the nitrosamines are the most important. To become carcinogenic these are metabolised by microsomal hydroxylases to form the alkyl diazohydroxide and then the methyl carbonium ion, which is the ultimate carcinogen.

Besides microsomal enzymes bacteria in the intestine may convert potential carcinogens to active cancer-inducing agents. One example is cycasin, a compound obtained from plants. Cycasin is methylazoxymethanol glucoside and if bacteria are present which contain a beta glucosidase enzyme they will liberate methylazoxymethanol, the carbonium ion of which is the ultimate carcinogen as it is for the synthetic carcinogen dimethylnitrosamine. The formation of such highly reactive electrophilic products by intestinal micro-organisms acting on substrates in the diet could be an important mechanism in the causation of cancer of the large intestine.

It would seem that the most important chemical carcinogens are highly reactive compounds. It also seems (p. 252) that two processes are involved, initiation and promotion. We can take these in turn.

There is now little doubt that in most cases initiation is in fact the production of mutations. This always seemed likely because the essence of a cancer is that the malignant change is passed on from one cell generation to the next by the genetic apparatus of the cell. Since we

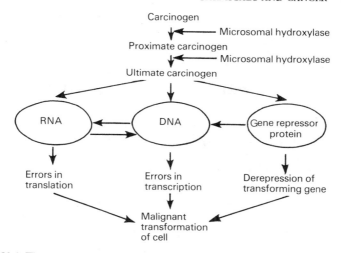

Fig. 39.1 The ways in which chemicals may induce cancer in body cells.

are dealing with somatic as opposed to germ cells we can say that much malignant disease is due to somatic mutation.

The proof of the mutagenicity of known human carcinogens such as beta-naphthylamine was established by what is commonly known as the Ames test, after its discoverer. A mutant strain of bacteria, usually *Salmonella typhimurium* is used, which is abnormal in that it cannot grow in the absence of histidine. Chemical mutagens reverse this bacterial mutation so that when they are added to the cultures the micro-organisms begin to grow. Most carcinogens failed to show mutagenesis until it was realised that they first had to be converted to the active ultimate carcinogens by microsomal hydroxylases. When this is done, by incubating the suspected substance with liver extract, before adding it to the bacterial culture, 90 per cent of chemical carcinogens are found to be mutagenic and 90 per cent of non-carcinogens are found to be non-mutagenic.

A figure for mutagenicity of 90 per cent is very high, considering the potential carcinogens in our environment and it has to be asked why even more people do not succumb to cancer. The reason may well lie in the variability of the microsomal hydroxylase system. There is considerable variation between individuals in the degree to which particular substances induce this enzyme system to become active. There is similar variation between different components of the enzyme system. In some individuals, the enzyme reactions leading to formation of mutagenic intermediates are stronger than those causing final detoxication (Fig. 39.2) and in others the situation is reversed.

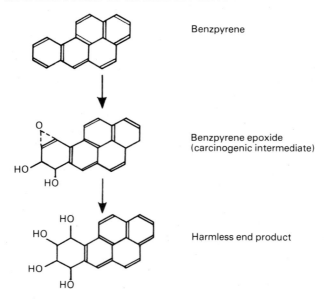

Fig. 39.2 The conversion of the polycyclic hydrocarbon, benzpyrene, to the carcinogenic intermediate, benzpyrene epoxide and eventually to a harmless metabolite, by the enzymic action of host tissue microsomal hydroxylases.

The molecular basis of the ability of carcinogens to cause somatic cell mutation is in most cases an intimate reaction with DNA. Some carcinogens link themselves directly to guanine as do polycyclic hydrocarbon epoxides. Some add methyl groups to guanine, some remove amino groups from cytosine and others cause cross links between the two chains of a DNA molecule.

These chemical alterations in DNA cause faulty pairing of bases to occur whenever DNA is replicated. For example, guanine which has been methylated is 'mistaken' for adenine so that when the affected DNA is replicated an A-T base pair is formed instead of the G-C base pair which was needed. When an epoxide is added directly to a guanine base, a massive distortion of the DNA molecule results with inevitable faulty replication.

In spite of these severe effects, chemical interference with DNA molecules by carcinogens is by no means always followed by cellular mutation. This is because cells have a battery of enzymes devoted to the excision and repair of faulty strands of DNA. It seems quite likely that somatic mutation and hence cancer, occurs only when the repair mechanism fails (perhaps because there was a mutation in the DNA which codes for it) or when the cell is forced into errors of DNA repair. It seems likely that it is faulty repair rather than the chemical reaction of mutagen and DNA, which is the direct cause of carcinogenic mutation. Errors in DNA repair are more likely to occur when the affected cells are dividing quickly rather than more slowly and this may be why cancer develops preferentially in organs where cell turnover is high, such as in the intestine rather than where it is low, for example in skeletal muscle.

Mutation can only occur when DNA is replicated, which means when the cell is dividing. Events such as faulty base pairing, leading to error-prone DNA repair, occur particularly during recombination. This is the process in which segments of DNA exchange with the corresponding segment on the other chromosome of the pair. Recombination during mitosis augments recruitment of fresh bases from the nuclear sap (p. 198) as a mechanism for mutation during cell division.

Mutation (alias initiation) is obviously crucial in understanding cancer but promotion also is important. The essence of promotion is accelerated cell division. It can be demonstrated experimentally that after administration of a mutagenic carcinogen, cancer follows more quickly if the skin is irritated or wounded, if the liver is forced to regenerate or if cell division in thyroid or ovary is accelerated by hormonal treatment. In humans, an increased risk of cancer is associated with ulcerative colitis, where the bowel epithelium regenerates excessively for many years, with exaggerated proliferation of the epithelium of the tongue, with irritation of the lip, with Paget's disease of the bone where bone cell turnover is much increased, or with the irritation caused by gall stones where the epithelium is again obliged to regenerate rapidly.

Why should excessive replication promote cancer in cell populations which are dividing rapidly anyway? Mutation (initiation) must precede promotion, so the effect has to be to augment the effects of mutation. The answer is not known. Hurried cell division could increase the chances of faulty DNA base repair. It could also increase the possibility of mistakes at cell division, so that a cell was left with two copies of a mutant gene instead of only one, by a kind of non-disjunction (p. 211) or as a result of exaggerated somatic recombination. Promotion could also be due to activation of latent genes which happen to have undergone carcinogenic mutation.

In contemplating the role of mutation and promotion in cancer in man one returns again and again to the phenomenon of latency. The daughters of mothers who received diethylstilboestrol during pregnancy did not develop cancer of the vagina until 16 to 19 years after their birth. The long latent periods associated with industrial cancer and cigarette smoking have already been mentioned.

Just as striking as latency is the extraordinary effect of ageing and the passage of time. The death rate from cancer of the large bowel rises 1000 fold between the ages of 30 and 80 years and this is typical of many other tumours. The combined effects of latency and the passing of years produce particularly complex graphs when the incidence of bronchial carcinoma in smokers, ex-smokers and non-smokers is plotted against the passage of time.

These various graphs and curves have been studied intensively by mathematicians. They are in virtual agreement that the observed facts can be explained only by accepting that malignant transformation occurs as the end result of a series of separate steps, taking place at different times, in the lifespan of an individual. This is known as the 'multiple hit' hypothesis. The most popular explanation is to assume that each cell contains n genes, each of which independently prevents cancer from developing. Only when all n genes are neutralised by separate mutations, does cancer arise. The chance of any single mutation occurring rises in direct proportion to our age, whether the mutation be 'spontaneous' or related to exposure to a carcinogen. Thus the likelihood of cancer will rise in direct proportion to age to the power of n. If the number of 'cancer restraining' genes is 4, then the risk of cancer would increase as the age to the power of 4. This means that the logarithm of cancer incidence should be linearly related to age which indeed in most cases it is. The slope for cancer of the large bowel indicates that $n = 6$, i.e. that 6 mutations are needed to bring about the disease.

Although mutation figures prominently in current thinking about chemical carcinogenesis we must not forget the possibility of non-genetic or epigenetic mechanisms. Chemical carcinogens react with RNA and gene repressor protein as well as with DNA. Reversion from malignancy occurs occasionally in real tumours as well as in the laboratory. Finally, malignancies can be induced by presumptive non-mutational mechanisms such as removing an organ from its normal hormonal control or by interfering with cell to cell communication by insertion of plastic sheets into the tissues.

Bibliography

Cairns J 1978 Cancer, science and society. Freeman, San Francisco

Coombs M M 1980 Chemical carcinogenesis: a view at the end of the first half-century. J. Path. 130: 117

di Paulo J A, Heidelberger C (eds) 1974) Chemical carcinogenesis. Dekker, New York

McCann Joyce, Choi E, Yamasaki Edith, Ames B N 1975 Detection of carcinogens as mutagens in the Salmonella/microsome test: assay of 300 chemicals. Proceedings of the National Academy of science, USA, 72: 5135

Magee P N 1973 In: Doll R A, Vodapija L (eds) Host environment interactions in the aetiology of cancer in man. IARC, Lyon

40

Hormones and cancer

Certain organs of the body respond to hormones such as oestrogens, testosterone or prolactin by hyperplasia and hypertrophy (p. 192). Two of these organs, the breast and the prostate, are commonly the site of cancer, breast tumours being the commonest malignancy in women and arguably the greatest single problem in cancer studies. In addition, both prostatic and breast cancers are well known to undergo regression if action is taken to withdraw the hormones which stimulate them. Thus many cases of breast cancer show improvement if the ovaries are removed and many patients with prostatic cancer can be cured by administration of female sex hormones. There is therefore a *prima facie* case that tumours of these organs are in some way caused by hormone action or dependent on hormones for their growth.

This hypothesis has been proved in the case of some tumours of animals. Mice of susceptible genetic strains receiving the Bittner mammary tumour virus in their mother's milk will not develop breast cancers if prolactin, oestrogen and progesterone are denied them by removing the pituitary, adrenals and ovaries. In the presence of the appropriate hormones all the mice will develop tumours. A similar situation holds for chemical carcinogens. Thus in some strains of rats, a single injection of a polycyclic hydrocarbon (dimethylbenzanthracene, DMBA) will induce breast tumours in 100 per cent of cases. If, however, the ovaries are removed, and also the adrenals or pituitary, the tumours do not occur and will disappear if already induced. Injection of oestrogens causes the tumours to recommence their growth unless the pituitary has been removed. This indicates that prolactin as well as oestrogen is necessary because it now seems almost certain that the contribution of the pituitary gland to mammary cancer is by secretion of the peptide hormone, prolactin. There is evidence also that oestrogens induce the release of prolactin from the pituitary gland and enhance its effect on breast tissue. There is also evidence that high levels of prolactin in the blood enhance the growth of mammary cancer only when oestrogens are present. The general conclusion is that prolactin, oestrogen and possibly progesterone are all necessary for the induction of mammary tumours by viral or chemical carcinogens.

In all these cases, the role of the hormones seems to be permissive, i.e. they permit carcinogenesis to occur rather than themselves cause it. This suggests that in the terms of the previous chapter, they are promotors rather than mutagens. On the other hand transplanting mouse ovaries to a site where they are inaccessible to normal hormonal control causes ovarian cancer to develop. This disappears when the ovary is replaced in its natural site. This seems to be one of the rare epigenetic cancers where mutation cannot be involved. It is however likely to be the exception rather than the rule and it is wiser to think of hormones as promoters rather than initiators of malignancy. It may be that in certain organs, hormones are essential for DNA synthesis even under carcinogenic stimulation. The effect of ovarian hormones on breast tissue is to increase the number of cells in mitosis rather than accelerate the rate of individual mitoses, i.e. shorten the cell cycle. The permissive role of these hormones is supported by work in which breast tissue in organ culture outside the body has been transformed to adenocarcinoma by DMBA but only in the presence of suitable amounts of oestrogen, prolactin and progesterone, the hormones themselves having no carcinogenic effect in this system.

Returning to the problem of breast cancer in women it has long been known that only some patients respond to hormone therapy such as ovariectomy. It was then realised that the hormone dependence of a particular tumour could be predicted by studying the pattern in the urine of the excretion products of various adrenal and ovarian hormones. More important, prospective epidemiological studies showed that women consistently excreting low amounts of aetiocholanalone (an androgen product) had a much higher risk of developing breast cancer than women excreting larger amounts. Another important clue comes from other studies also using a combined epidemiological and endocrine approach. These showed that women with a high rate of breast cancer had in their urine a low ratio of oestriol (E3) to the other metabolites of oestrogen, i.e. oestrone (E1) and oestradiol (E2). Conversely, women with a low rate of breast cancer had a high ratio of E3 to E1 and E2. Although it is not easy to produce neoplasia in animals with oestrogens alone, E1 and E2 can be shown to have carcinogenic potential, whereas E3 does not and may even inhibit tumour formation. It would appear therefore that preferential conversion of oestrogen to E1 and E2 as opposed to the less carcinogenic E3 may be a causative or permissive factor in cancer of the breast and that low production of the androgen metabolite aetiocholanalone may have a similar effect.

The incidence of breast cancer varies greatly from one part of the world to another. Many factors have been suggested to explain these differences. It now seems clear that the most important single determinant is the age at which women have their first child. Women producing a first full-time baby before they are 18 years old have one-third of the risk of developing breast cancer of women becoming pregnant after the age of 35 years. So far, age of onset of first pregnancy correlates as predicted with the oestriol ratios described above. It would seem that having a baby at an early age has a permanent effect on oestrogen (and possibly androgen) metabolism which confers a high degree of protection against breast cancer throughout life. The question is, protection against what? The answer is unknown; oncogenic virus, other hormones such as oestradiol, environmental carcinogens, and dietary habits have all been suggested. As regards the latter, E.G. Knox has shown a very close correlation between the proportion of the diet taken as fat and the risk of mammary carcinoma. In the meantime, the incidence of breast cancer in the Western world is rising.

Bibliography

Doll R, Vadopija L (eds) 1973) Host environment interactions in the aetiology of cancer in man (Especially articles by McMahon B, Pearson O H and Shapiro S) IARC, Lyon

Vorherr H et al 1978 Breast cancer: potentially predisposing and protecting factors. Role of pregnancy, lactation and endocrine status. Amer. J. Obst. gynaecology 130: 335

41

Other causes of cancer

Ionising radiation

There is unequivocal evidence that electromagnetic radiation e.g. ultraviolet light and X-rays and particulate radiation, e.g. electrons, neutrons and α particles causes cancer in man (Table 41.1). The most important is ultraviolet light because it is probably the commonest cause of skin cancer. The evidence here, as in the case of cigarettes and lung cancer, is epidemiological. It comes from a statistical association between UV irradiation on the one hand and cancer of exposed lightly

Table 41.1 Agents known to produce cancer in man

Agent	Site of cancer
Various polycyclic hydrocarbons	Scrotum
Ionizing radiation	Skin, bronchus, marrow and most if not all organs
Ultraviolet light	Skin
2-naphthylamine	
1-naphthylamine	Bladder
Benzidine	
Asbestos	Bronchus, pleura and peritoneum
'Chrome ore'	Bronchus
'Nickel ore'	Bronchus, nasal sinuses
Bischloromethyl ether	Bronchus
Hardwood dust (?)	Nasal sinuses
'Isopropyl oil'	Nasal sinuses
Benzene	Marrow
'Betel mixture'	Mouth
Chlornaphazine (treatment of myeloma)	Bladder
Arsenic (when used as medicine)	Skin, bronchus
Phenacetin (in study of analgesic nephropathy)	Renal pelvis
Tobacco	Bronchus: also mouth, pharynx, larynx, oesophagus, bladder
Mustard gas	Bronchus, larynx, nasal sinuses
Vinyl chloride	Angiosarcoma of the liver
Stilboestrol	Male breast, vagina in child exposed in utero
Aflatoxin	Liver

pigmented parts of the skin on the other. Thus skin cancer is much commoner in the sunny southern states of the USA than in the North but rare in the black population. UV light will induce skin tumours in animals and will provoke mutations in many forms of life in direct proportion to its ability to cause tumours. This suggests that it launches a direct attack on the genetic apparatus and it has indeed been confirmed that UV irradiation forms bonds between adjacent bases in nuclear DNA with formation of abnormal thymine dimers. It is a reasonable assumption that this deformation of DNA leads to malignant transformation. The best evidence for this cause and effect relationship comes from a rare, genetically determined disease called xeroderma pigmentosa. The genetic abnormality is lack of an enzyme which normally repairs defects in nuclear DNA. Patients with the disease have an extremely high incidence of skin cancer in those parts of the body exposed to sunlight. The inference is that UV irradiation regularly causes defects in cell DNA in the skin, that these abnormalities are normally repaired by a specific enzyme system but that if the enzyme is lacking or inadequate, or overwhelmed by the extent of DNA damage, then skin cancer results.

In the absence of xeroderma pigmentosa, the excision repair of dimers is virtually perfect. If by chance, two dimers are formed on opposite DNA chains and overlap, the repair mechanism fails and mutation will occur. Since this is a double event, its likelihood will increase as the square of the dose of UV irradiation. In other cases, irradiation induces an error-prone repair enzyme incapable of excising single dimers so that mutation occurs in direct proportion to the dose.

Radioactive emissions (Ch. 27) such as X-irradiation are well known as potent carcinogens. Many of the early pioneers, including Roentgen, developed skin cancer. Miners engaged in the excavation and extraction (and therefore inhalation) of radioactive ores, such as uranium, had a very high rate of bronchial carcinoma even in the pre-cigarette era when the disease was rare. Workers licking brushes dipped in radium-containing paint used for luminous watch dials, developed cancer of the jaw. Cancer of the bone marrow was common amongst early radiologists and the therapeutic use of even smallish doses of X-rays for a variety of diseases was frequently followed many years later by cancer in the treated part, e.g. in the thyroid gland. All these examples date from the days before the hazard was realised, but the survivors of the atomic bomb explosions in Japan had 5 to 10 years later, an incidence of bone marrow cancer about 15 times higher than non-irradiated control populations.

Forms of radiation other than UV light cause mutation by breaking chemical bonds in DNA rather than by forming new bonds. It is possible that those breaks are due to the formation within the cell of very active free radicles derived, for example, from intracellular water.

X-rays are relatively weak and cause single chain breaks which are easily repaired. As with UV light, mutation probably occurs only when two such breaks occur simultaneously and the repair mechanism fails. Because this demands two independent events, cancer-inducing mutation increases with the square of the dose of X-rays.

In the case of high energy particles such as neutrons, a single interaction with the particle will cause two DNA breaks which cannot, therefore, be repaired. As a result the mutation rate increases in direct proportion to the dose.

These predictions have been grimly fulfilled. The Nagasaki bomb produced mostly X-rays and the subsequent incidence of leukaemia was proportional to the square of the calculated dose received by the patient. The Hiroshima bomb produced a heavy output of neutrons and the subsequent leukaemia incidence was proportional directly to the dose received.

Although radioactivity-induced cancer is evidently dose-dependent, it cannot truly be said that there is a safe lower threshold of response. A study of workers at the nuclear submarine base at Rosyth showed chromosome defects in direct proportion to exposure to gamma rays. In particular, aberrations were found at levels of exposure well below the internationally agreed occupational and environmental maximal permissible limits. These aberrations were unstable and therefore presumably repairable, but presumably the chance of a 'double hit', even at permissible doses does exist.

Genetic factors

Some aspects of the role of inheritance in causing cancer have been discussed in Chapter 31. Examples of tumours due to simple gene inheritance and showing Mendelian transmission through the generations are scarce. The two most important are retinoblastoma, an autosomal dominant occurring in children and polyposis coli. The latter starts as multiple benign tumours which then become malignant in adult life. They are often quoted as examples of benign tumours acquiring malignant characteristics, but should probably be seen as cancer which gets off to a slow start. Genetically determined malignancies would be expected to eliminate themselves by natural selection since most sufferers would die before producing children and this probably explains their relative rarity. The two exceptions quoted above may be attributable to a high mutation rate in the affected genes or, in the case of polyposis coli to a relatively delayed onset.

Whereas single gene defects are rare, polygenic inheritance is probably important in the causation of cancer. Polygenic inheritance in this instance means that the total parcel of inherited genetic information favours the operation of environmental carcinogens on a particular organ. Cancer of the breast is not inherited and is probably due to viral, chemical or hormonal causes (p. 259), but is three times more frequent in the daughters or sisters of mammary cancer patients than in the general populace. In man, there are many other cancers which show a definite but modest predilection for affected families. By contrast, bronchial and bladder carcinoma show no familial trend. There is never an inherited tendency to develop cancer in general, as opposed to cancer at a particular site.

It is important not to confuse environmental factors with inherited ones. Many cancers are commoner in social class V, e.g. gastric carcinoma, and so may appear to cluster in families who remain impoverished over several generations. Others may be related to occupations which tend to stay in the family, such as the tendency of publicans to develop carcinoma of the oesophagus.

Although genetic factors may not be of paramount importance in practical terms, they throw light on the role of mutation in carcinogenesis and provide suport for the 'multiple hit' hypothesis. There is a tumour called a neuroblastoma which may occur early in childhood and be inherited as a monogenic Mendelian dominant or occur in adult life without apparent genetic determination. Bilateral neuroblastoma is more likely to occur early and be obviously inherited than a unilateral tumour. This situation fits best with the view that the neuroblastoma mutation may occur both in the germ cell and in the somatic cell and that at least two mutations ('hits') are needed to produce a tumour. A 'hit' in the germ cell followed by a second mutation leads to the tumour. The second 'hit' may be in the germ cell, in which case the tumour appears early in life, or may be somatic in which case the tumour will devlop later. Bilateral tumours imply homozygocity of the mutation and hence are highly heritable. In non-genetic cases of neuroblastoma all mutations are thought to be somatic with none in the germ cells and hence the tumour does not develop until adult life. It is of interest that the incidence of genetically determined neuroblastoma is the same in Japan as it is in the USA. This similarity in incidence compares sharply with the great differences which exist in environmentally determined cancers (p. 273).

Breast cancer shows some analogies with this complex situation. A woman with cancer in one breast is three times more likely than an unaffected control to have an affected first degree relative, but if the tumour is bilateral the figure rises to 8 times the control population risk. In familial polyposis coli it is believed that three mutations occur;

the first in the germ cell, inherited as an autosomal dominant, the second a somatic mutation in early life giving rise to the actual polyps and a third occurring around the age of 30 years and leading to the emergence of invasive cancer.

In addition to supporting the multiple mutation hypothesis of carcinogenesis, rare genetic cancers also buttress the view that failure of DNA repair is a central feature of malignancy (p. 256). There are several rare inherited diseases known as chromosomal breakage syndromes where autosomal chromosomes are aberrant and DNA repair is defective. One of these, xeroderma pigmentosa has already been discussed (p. 263). Others are Blooms syndrome, Fanconi anaemia and ataxia telangectasia. All are associated with a high cancer risk in a variety of organs. In Turner's syndrome (p. 213) there is a high risk of ovarian cancer, in Klinefelter's syndrome, of male breast cancer and in Down's syndrome, of chronic myeloid leukaemia. In this latter disease (CML) a specific chromosomal defect occurs in most cases involving a translocation between chromosomes 22 and 9, giving the so-called Philadelphia chromosome (Ph'). In Burkitt lymphoma (p. 246) there is a specific abnormality involving chromosome 14. All these examples strengthen the case for multiple mutation and faulty DNA repair as the essential elements in carcinogenesis. Familial cancer is seen in this light as occurring when the first mutation affects germinal, as opposed to somatic cells.

Chronic irritation

This is often given as a predisposing cause of cancer but the concept does not sustain close scrutiny. The smoking of clay pipes with hot stems or the practice of some tribes of holding hot dishes to the bare abdomen over long periods of time result in skin cancer of the lip and abdomen respectively and have been attributed to chronic irritation. Other examples of prolonged irritation and stimulation of cell renewal have been given on p. 257. The most likely explanation of these associations as set out on p. 257, is that they act as 'promotors' increasing the chance that somatic mutation in the affected cells will lead to malignant transformation.

Bibliography

Chromosomes in radiation-exposed workers 1979 Lancet 1: 453
Purtillo D T, Paquin Louise, Gindhart T 1978 Genetics of neoplasia. American Journal of Pathology 91: 607
Warren S 1970 Radiation carcinogenesis. New York Academy of Science 46: 133

42

Cancer and immunity

Previous chapters described how tumours induced by chemicals or viruses or occurring spontaneously from unknown causes acquire on the surface of their constituent cells new, tumour specific antigens (TSA) not present in normal tissues. Because these antigens are exposed on the cell surface, because they are alien and because the body's defences have not been previously exposed to them, they should illicit an immune response. This prediction is based largely on experience with the rejection of tissue grafts such as skin or kidney when the graft has surface (histocompatibility) antigens which differ from those of the recipient. The concept that tumours are immunogenic is supported by numerous demonstrations in patients of circulating antibodies or sensitised lymphocytes directed against their own tumours. Malignant melanoma seems to be particularly effective in this respect but many other types of cancer have been shown to produce similar effects.

The efficiency with which foreign tissue grafts are destroyed has led to suggestions that the speedy reaction to alien histo-compatibility antigens has evolved as a survival mechanism directed against the emergence of cancer cells. It is suggested that a continuous process of immunosurveillance exists in which circulating lymphocytes monitor the tissues for such antigens and destroy the intruding cells once a large enough clone of sensitised lymphocytes has been produced by initial contact with the antigen. The corollary of this hypothesis is that cancer would develop very much more frequently were it not for the apparatus of immunity. As we will see later, this hypothesis looks particularly shaky at the moment.

The rejection of skin grafts can be prevented if the immune defences are rendered ineffective. In theory therefore experimentally induced tumours should be initiated more readily in animals without an intact immune apparatus. In practice the incidence of tumours induced in experimental animals by viruses is greatly enhanced if immunosuppression is first performed by removing the thymus in early life or by injecting antilymphocyte serum. The incidence reverts to normal if immune lymphocytes are transfused to the affected animals, so is not due to an increased rate of transformation but rather to destruction of already transformed cells. The effect appears to be due mainly to lymphocytes of thymic origin, i.e. T cells (p. 38). A similar fall in tumour incidence has been observed after lymphocyte transfusion to animals in which cancer was induced by X-rays. On the whole, immunosuppression produces much less dramatic effects on the incidence of tumours induced by chemical carcinogens. It would seem in general that the more strongly antigenic is the tumour the more susceptible it is to immunological destruction.

Skin graft rejection can be accelerated by prior sensitisation of the animal to the graft antigens. Following our analogy, it is gratifying to find that the incidence of experimentally induced viral tumours can be reduced by prior sensitisation with a sample of the tumour cells. Indeed, a similar effect can by achieved in some viral and chemically provoked tumours by non-specific stimulation of the immune system by injection of various vaccines, especially BCG.

However, specific immunisation, although often effective if given before tumour induction, hardly ever affects the growth of established malignancies. Even more important is the discovery that in some cases, previous specific immunisation with cancer cells may actually enhance the growth of the tumour from which the cells were derived, when the tumour is transplanted into the immunised animal.

This brings us to the main conceptual problem of the immune control of cancer, namely the failure of the immune system to destroy clinical cancer more effectively than it appears to do. It is hard to invoke the analogy of a rapid overwhelming bacterial infection because we know that tumours must begin as only a few malignant cells and take some time to establish themselves. They must therefore be less immunogenic than we have postulated or successful in provoking some diversion of the immune response which prevents their destruction.

Although some tumours are indeed more antigenic than others there is ample evidence for the second suggestion. It has been shown that whereas it is cellular immunity, i.e. sensitised lymphocytes and macrophages which kills tumour cells, tumours also cause circulating antibody to be formed. This antibody forms complexes with the tumour antigens and in some way not understood these complexes prevent the immunological destruction of the tumours by lymphocytes and macrophages. The antibody is called blocking antibody and its presence may explain tumour enhancement by prior sensitisation. It is also possible that the mere formation of antibody may so occupy the immune apparatus as to prevent the arming of the lymphocytes and macrophages.

Another possible explanation of the lack of success of the immune response against cancer is provided by *in vitro* experiments in which small numbers of sensitised lymphocytes were found to stimulate tumour growth whereas large numbers inhibited the tumour cells. The mechanism is unknown but the phenomenon can be reproduced *in vivo*. It would seem that a combination of a large tumour with a normal immune response or of a small tumour with a weak or slow immune response leads to enhancement of tumour growth instead of suppression. The problem remains of why early tumours should arouse only a weak response. One explanation is that they tend to arise in privileged sites, i.e. areas of the body where even foreign antigens fail to provoke an immune response. Thus in the mouse, the mammary gland is a privileged site and a tumour growing there becomes immunogenic only when it extends beyond the confines of the mammary fat pad. By this time, of course, it is too large to be susceptible to immunological attack. The same may be true of human breast cancer and also of many other epithelial tumours.

Finally, since tumours or individual tumour cells vary in their antigenicity, it seems inevitable that if immunodestruction is partially effective, a process of natural selection will lead to preferential growth of tumour cells of low antigenicity. Similarly, if immunoenhancement were predominant, natural selection would favour those tumour cells responding best to immunostimulation at the expense of those susceptible to immunodestruction. In either case the tumour could be predicted to adjust its antigenicity to the level best suited for its continued growth, and incidentally for the death of its host, the patient.

It can be seen that there is no shortage of excuses for the failure of the immune system to eliminate malignant tumours in spite of their alien antigens. The concept of immune surveillance, i.e. that tumours are prevented from developing by an intact immune system has, however, received a severe blow following the realisation that patients with grossly impaired immunity are not in general more likely than others to develop cancer. The striking exception to this rule is malignancy of the lymphoid tissue itself (lymphoma) which is indeed much more common in immunodeficient patients. The evidence comes both from patients whose immune system has been artificially depressed to allow the acceptance of kidney grafts and from those born with defective immunity of various sorts.

Taking these observations on patients together with the experimental findings discussed above it would seem that immunity is effective mainly against virus-induced tumours and against tumours of the lymphoid system. It is particularly ineffective against most cancers of man. As we have seen, there are many possible explanations of this latter inadequacy. It is also possible, if one so wishes, to conclude that with the exception of the lymphomas, human malignant tumours appear more likely to be due to chemical carcinogens than to oncogenic viruses.

Bibliography

Baldwin R W 1974 In: Ts'o P.O.P, Di paolo J A (Eds) Chemical carcinogenesis, part B. Dekker, New York
Green I, Cohen S, McClusky R T 1977 Mechanisms of tumor immunity. Wiley, New York
Mitchison N A, Makela O 1973 In: Doll R, Vodopija L (eds) Host environment interactions in the aetiology of cancer in man. LIARC, Lyon
Stoll B A (ed) 1975 Host defense in breast cancer. Heinemann, London

43

Epidemiology of cancer

All advances in cancer studies in man seem to come initially from an observation concerning the incidence of a particular tumour in a particular population. Scrotal cancer in chimney sweeps of the eighteenth and nineteenth centuries, bladder cancer in workers in the aniline dye industry, bronchial cancer in cigarette smokers, skin cancer in X-ray pioneers, mesothelioma in asbestos workers, Burkitt lymphoma in inhabitants of East Africa are all examples of how an alert observer can open a door to fresh understanding of the cancer problem.

The interpretation of epidemiological data can be very difficult. Cancer of the cervix of the uterus is much less common in Jewish women than in other members of the population and this led to the speculation that circumcision of the sexual partner was a protective factor. This would seem to be borne out by the lower incidence of the disease in the circumcised Moslems of Yugoslavia than in the non-Moslem population of the same country. However, cloistered nuns have a very low incidence of cervical cancer as do Seventh Day Adventists. There is also in many countries a strong inverse correlation with socio-economic group, the lowest income group having the highest incidence. Cluster analysis of all these sets of figures revealed two factors which seemed to spell a high risk of cervical cancer and which seemed to cut across all other apparent group affinities. The two factors are an early age at first sexual intercourse and a high number of sexual partners and they operate largely regardless of race, religion, circumcision or economic status.

The association of cervical cancer with frequent intercourse with many sexual partners from an early age suggests the operation of a sexually transmitted infective agent, most effective if introduced when the patient is young. Herpes virus II is sexually transmitted and patients with cervical cancer usually have much higher levels of antibody to this virus in their blood than do matched controls. There is a good chance that this DNA virus, which is similar to that associated with Burkitt lymphoma, may be proven to be a major factor in the cause of cervical cancer. If so, it will be the epidemiologists who led the virologists to their goal.

One of the most fascinating and important aspects of the cancer problem is the enormous differences that exist between the frequency of occurrence of particular tumours in different parts of the world (Fig. 43.1). Liver cancer is common in the Bantu of Southern Africa, but rare in the black population of the USA of Bantu origin and it was concluded 30 years ago that this must mean that an environmental factor was responsible not a racial one. Indeed, the vast majority of geographical differences in cancer rates are due to environmental features which in theory could be identified and neutralised. This is another way of saying that most cancer is potentially preventable if the clues presented by epidemiology are followed. Where clear-cut racial factors operate they seem to be protective, as in the rarity of cancer of the testis in the Congo-Kordofamian group whether resident in Africa, the USA or the West Indies.

Risk differentials can be used to find out if patients with a particular cancer have things in common, whether they live in areas of high or low frequency of that cancer. Thus cases of bronchial carcinoma occurring in either a high risk or a low risk area anywhere in the world show a close correlation with cigarette smoking. The conclusion is that in the low risk regions, either fewer people smoke, or that they smoke less dangerous cigarettes, or that other things make smoking less carcinogenic than elsewhere.

There are great differences in the geographical incidence of breast cancer and studies in the UK, USA, Brazil, Japan, Greece, Yugoslavia and Taiwan have shown that much of this variation relates to the age of first pregnancy. In other words, pregnancy at an early age confers a high degree of protection against some other causative factor, for example, an RNA oncogenic virus. Lactation practices such as the duration of breast feeding, once thought to be important, seem to be irrelevant.

Japan is a magnet for cancer epidemiologists. Apart from the low incidence of breast cancer there is also the striking rarity of cancer of the prostate and equally marked frequency of cancer of the stomach compared with western countries. Both these differentials are as yet unexplained.

Some other geographical differences, especially in the incidence of skin cancer, such as its frequency in Australia, are easily explained by exposure to sunlight. Other geographical risk differentials are quite bizarre. In the Caspian Littoral of Iran there is a dramatic gradient in the incidence of oesophageal cancer with differences up to 20 fold between the Eastern and Western ends of the coast line. The risk of

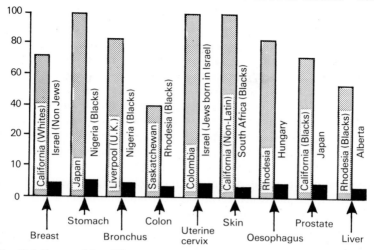

Fig. 43.1 Some striking differences between incidence rates of particular cancers in different parts of the world (Modified from R. Doll).

oesophageal cancer seems to correlate with the rainfall, the lowest rainfall being associated with the highest incidence. Rainfall may determine vegetation and therefore diet.

Of particular use in establishing the importance of environmental factors has been the study of migrant populations. When Japanese with a very high rate of gastric cancer migrate to the U.S.A. they at first retain their high incidence. With the next generation of U.S. born Japanese, however, the incidence falls dramatically, even when all marriages are within the original Japanese ethnic group. Conversely, Japanese with a low rate of large bowel cancer acquire the high incidence of the U.S. population after migration to that country. These observations and others make it quite plain that some environmental factor, probably dietary habits, and not a genetic determinant is responsible for the differential incidence of these forms of cancer, since the risk correlates with the environment and customs and not with race. Breast cancer in Japanese migrants to the U.S.A. also shows an increased incidence compared with the low levels in Japan, but the increase is slower and less dramatic than in the case of cancer of the large bowel.

The relationship of cancer to age also provides important information. In general, tumours become much more frequent as one gets older but there are exceptions and amendments to this principle. The most obvious is the case of tumours of childhood, some of which are due to genetic determinants, e.g. retinoblastoma. Another pattern is a progressive incidence with age, slowing down after middle age as occurs in cancer of the breast or uterine cervix. Another type of age-incidence curve is typified by bronchial carcinoma and shows a peak in late middle age followed by some decline in incidence. Finally, some tumours such as gastric cancer show a steady, uninterrupted increase in incidence from adolescence to old age.

In all these last three instances, statistical analysis shows the relationship of incidence with age to be due not to ill-defined ageing processes, or to increased spontaneous somatic mutation, or to loss of potency by the immunity system, but to a greater or less exposure to environmental carcinogens. In gastric cancer we can conclude that the longer we live the more the exposure. The break in the curve of bronchial carcinoma is due to the relatively sudden increase in the popularity of cigarettes affecting only certain cohorts of the populace. In other words the very old acquired the habit of cigarette smoking too late in life to influence the cause of their death. Breast and cervical cancer can be presumed to be due to factors to which we are exposed less and less after a certain age. In cancer of the cervix there is no problem in explaining this declining risk (p. 271). Cancer of the breast remains an enigma. The relationship of cancer to socio-economic status is complex. Within a fairly homogeneous culture such as the UK. or U.S.A, almost all cancers are more common in the less affluent and less well educated. There are many reasons for this, such as smoking habits, dietary and drinking patterns and exposure to industrial carcinogens. Taking the world as a whole, the inverse relationship between affluence and individual cancers is not always present. Carcinoma of the large bowel shows a linear correlation between its age-corrected incidence and indices of prosperity, notably the proportion of the diet taken as beef. It would seem that the more beef one eats, the greater the risk of cancer of the colon. It must be admitted however that although the hypothesis is attractive, the real correlation may be with other cultural indices.

The striking differences in the relationship of cancer to occupation, habits, geography and age all emphasise that the great majority of tumours are due to environmental factors which are theoretically identifiable and preventable. For the most part, these environmental factors consist of dietary practices, social customs, habits such as smoking and of exposure to industrial processes. We are, therefore, talking mainly of a micro-environment which, except for the constraints of poverty, men may abandon or retain as they wish.

Bibliography

Cairns J 1978 Cancer, science and society. Freeman, San Francisco
Doll R, Vodopija L (eds) 1973 Host environment interactions in the aetiology of cancer in man (especially articles by Muir C S, Roll R, Shapiro S) IARC, Lyon

44

Psychopathology

In both general and specialised medical practice, a high proportion of patients who come seeking help are not suffering from any demonstrable physical abnormality although they may have symptoms such as abdominal pain, headache, insomnia or loss of appetite which suggest bodily disease. These patients are categorised as having functional illness and if their complaints are persistent and not merely a temporary reaction to personal setbacks, their illness is usually classified as neurosis.

Neurotics are a different group from those with psychosomatic illness where activity of the autonomic nervous system, due to emotional disturbance, causes or aggravates symptoms which form definite patterns, and where structural change is demonstrable in the affected organs, usually the gastrointestinal tract. Although it is convenient to make this distinction, the two sets of patients do admittedly have many features in common.

The bodily symptoms of neurosis may seem real enough to the patients, but they originate in the mind, and as well as complaining of illness which simulates organic pathology they commonly suffer from disabilities which are purely emotional or mental, e.g. feelings of sadness or unworthiness, unjustifiable anxiety or tension or inability to concentrate. They may exhibit compulsive behaviour patterns which make them miserable or may get them into trouble with the police. Psychiatrists apply a variety of labels to these sufferers of which depression is currently most in vogue and anxiety states and hysteria also popular. For the purposes of this brief discussion we can use the term 'neurosis' to cover them all.

Besides all these patients there are those termed psychotic or insane. Some of these have delusions or hallucinations and exhibit bizarre thought patterns. Others are intensely excited at times, suicidally depressed at others. Some believe themselves to be persecuted and cannot be persuaded otherwise. These disorders are usually termed schizophrenia, manic depressive illness and paranoia respectively.

The disturbances we have been describing originate in consciousness and subconsciousness and these functions reside in the brain. It is natural to ask whether disease of the type discussed in all the other chapters of this book could affect the brain so as to produce these symptoms. From the fact that Freud himself asked this question and then went on to discover subconscious motivation, repressed instincts, childhood sexuality and psychoanalysis we can conclude that in general the answer is no. Some organic diseases of the nervous system produce symptoms such as loss of memory or judgement although they rarely show symptoms of depression or schizophrenia. An especially important example is dementia, which is a common feature of senility (senile dementia). Demented patients are confused as to space and time and may well have specific delusions, e.g. about their identity. Atherosclerosis of the cerebral vessels and cerebral anoxia may be important factors and can sometimes be successfully relieved by vascular by-pass surgery. In other cases irreversible neurone loss seems to be the cause. Dementia also occurs in presenile patients, e.g. young adults and may be due to slow virus infection. Porphyria, liver and kidney failure are other causes of dementia but it also occurs in the course of acute infections such as pneumonia. Intense efforts have been made to establish a pathological basis for the psychoses, especially schizophrenia. When morbid anatomy failed to provide an answer, attention was directed to disturbed metabolism especially of amino acids or catecholamines. Many hypotheses have been launched but all have foundered. Currently there is much interest in a possible genetic basis for schizophrenia which could be polygenic and even monogenic but with low penetrance.

There is also much excitement concerning the endorphins, which are opiate-like peptides produced within the body and which act on cerebral receptors. These remarkable endogenous compounds can influence thresholds of perceived pain and their release by appropriate stimulation may be the organic basis of the anaesthesia produced by acupuncture. There have been many suggestions that they may have a more general role in thinking and feeling and not unexpectedly have been involved in the pathogenesis of mental illness, especially schizophrenia. As yet the evidence is unconvincing.

In neuroses there have been even more intensive efforts. There have for example been many attempts to show that depression was due to a disequilibrium in the levels of certain catecholamines in the brain, but again without convincing results. In spite of this failure there is no doubt that certain drugs have made the management of these illnesses much easier. Chlorpromazine makes the schizophrenic much less agitated and amenable to reason, diazepam calms the anxious neurotic and the tricyclic drugs or monoamine oxidase inhibitors elevate the mood of the depressive. In some ways it would seem as if we are back in the days of Jenner, when vaccines prevented smallpox before men knew the cause of the disease or even that bacteria, let alone viruses, existed.

On the other hand we have the enormous body of evidence linking the traumas of early childhood with neurosis and demonstrating the powerful influence of suppressed emotions in shaping neurotic symptoms. Psychiatrists who are enthusiastic supporters of the biochemical view of mental illness will, when they treat their patients, always combine the use of psychomotor drugs with psychotherapy based more or less on theories of subconscious motivation.

Looking at this confused situation it seems reasonable to reconcile the conflicting evidence by suggesting that three factors are at work; the events which are impinging on the patient's present life, the events which took place in childhood which are now repressed in the subconscious mind and his mood level or personality type. With regard to this third factor we could say that anxiety corresponds to fear and timidity in the personality; depression to pessimism and guilt; and paranoia to suspicion and aggression. The schizophrenic personality is withdrawn, uncommunicative and sensitive.

All these personality traits are normal variations of human types. It is probable that they are determined by a mixture of genetic and environmental factors. It is also probable that they determine which type of mental disturbance will develop when circumstances favour its onset. The circumstances which have this precipitating effect we can summarise as Freudian (meaning all repressed subsconscious emotions and reactions) and the stresses of everyday life. Since psychomotor drugs affect mood level probably by regulating catecholamine metabolism in the brain, it is reasonable to suppose that they work on the cerebral background to neurosis by controlling intensity of anxiety, depression and excitement without affecting subconscious or environmental factors. Psychotherapy deals with the repressed emotive forces and counselling, common sense and understanding with the environmental forces.

This analysis forces us to ask whether mental disturbance has any place at all in the subject matter of pathology since repressed emotions and impulses, variable personality traits and problems of adjustment to life, are all part of normal existence. There are several reasons for asking this question. There is as yet no substantial pathogenic basis for these maladies, the distinction between normality and abnormality is largely subjective, psychiatric symptoms are often vital defensive stratagems, the diagnosis depends as much on cultural criteria as on medical judgement and the dividing line between malingering and neurosis can sometimes be very blurred.

The dubious nature of mental illness has been taken up by one psychiatrist in particular. Szasz suggests that what we term mental illness represents a withdrawal from the harsh realities of life and is often a form of game playing in which attempts are made to coerce others to do as the patient wants. Our culture accepts illness as an excuse for rejecting the everyday responsibilities of life such as earning a living, the care of dependents or mature relationships with others. In harsher cultures illness is concealed lest the sufferer be denied opportunities for obtaining food due to his disability. It is obvious that in our culture some of those who have no physical pathology, but who feel the need to escape responsibilities, or feel unable to cope with them, will develop symptoms which simulate illness. When this is done consciously it is called malingering. When done unconsciously it is called neurosis or hysteria. When reality is denied without insight it is called psychosis.

In times when medical awareness was less widespread, neurosis usually took the form of physical symptoms such as bizarre paralyses. Nowadays, subjective, less easily demolished symptoms like headache, fatigue, palpitations, insomnia are more common. Psychotic symptoms such as irrational and inappropriate behaviour, hallucinations and delusions can also be seen as a means of withdrawal from unpleasant reality in favour of a self-created world. The symptoms of neurosis may seem more unpleasant than the real-life situation of the patient. We must accept, however, that the conflict between reality on the one hand and the patient's personality and unconscious instincts on the other may be very intense and threatening to the patient. Symptoms represent an attempt to resolve these conflicts, e.g. by transferring anxiety about a repressed forbidden urge to some external situation, as in claustrophobia. In addition, they can be used as weapons in coercive game playing and by making the patient ill they help to ensure him some protection from external pressures and give him the privileged status of a patient.

In the case of the most frequent psychiatric diagnosis, depression or affective disorder as it is also known, there is particular controversy between those who regard it as a biochemical imbalance and others who see it as a reaction to sadistic and masochistic impulses repressed in childhood. As with most controversies in pathology it seems likely that time will show both parties to have glimpsed part of the truth, since the best treatment is usually a combination of psychomotor drugs and psychotherapy. Depressive illness seems almost to be reaching epidemic proportions and one of the main preoccupations of. physicians is deciding whether a patient is depressed or justifiably unhappy. Careful study shows that real depression is almost always characterised by strong feelings of unworthiness. Rejection and failure or guilt-provoking stimuli such as criminal accusations or threatening letters from income tax inspectors, reinforce this feeling of unworthiness and may lead to suicide. On the other hand, success and acclaim thought to be unjustified conflict strongly with the patient's secret view of himself and may produce an even more severe mental breakdown with intense anxiety and anguish which may again lead to suicide. It is not hard to think of celebrated suicides which fit these factors.

Some depressive states respond so dramatically to specific drugs such as lithium or monoamine oxadase inhibitors that they must be regarded as mainly if not enterely biochemical in origin. Similarly, depression which is merely part of a complex neurotic behaviour pattern may result purely from psychic conflicts. The apparent increase in the incidence of affective disorder makes one suspect also that cultural changes may be important. Perhaps the increased intensity of parental support conflicts so strongly with the realities of life subsequently encountered, that feelings of unworthiness inevitably arise. Depressive illness shows a strong familial tendency which does not seem to fit very well with conventional genetics. Some of the familial pattern could well reflect parental attitudes which tend to be repeated from one generation to the next.

Depression also fits well into the views of those who hold most mental upsets to be pseudo-illnesses. In our society it is better to be labelled sick than lazy, criminal, irresponsible or inadequate and people who are fed up with the lack of satisfaction in their jobs, marriages or lives in general may welcome a psychiatric diagnosis because it transfers the responsibility for ordering their lives from themselves to others. This view point, as advanced for example by Ilich certainly has some validity. However, even in these cases some disability exists and exhortations are seldom helpful. The physician has no choice but to accept the individual at his own valuation as someone who is ill, and to treat the disability. He may, however, do so by declining the gambit of illness and instead help the patient to understand and to cope with his problems. The physician does not have the right to refuse involvement on the grounds that no genuine illness is present. He does, however, have the right and perhaps the duty to draw attention to those aspects of society which seem particularly likely to drive essentially stable people to seek the role of patient.

Bibliography

Ilich I 1974 Medical nemesis. Boyar
Szasz T 1972 The myth of mental illness. Paladin
Woodruff R A, Goodwin D W, Gotz S B 1974 Psychiatric diagnosis. Oxford University Press

45

Social pathology

Everybody knows that disease is caused by ignorance, overcrowding, poverty, malnutrition and filth and that much of the world's population is still in the grip of these agents. They also know that high living standards and efficient public health eradicate rickets, plague, typhus, cholera, typhoid, puerperal fever and tuberculosis. They also know that the same high standards of living have caused a crop of different diseases such as obesity and coronary thrombosis. The analysis of workers such as McKeown have made it very clear that almost all the extraordinary increase in life expectancy that occured in the British Isles between the seventeenth and early twentieth centuries was due to social change rather than advances in medical science or pathology. The contribution of these latter factors has been much more recent. Even the introduction of antibiotics and chemotherapy has had a minor effect on diseases such as tuberculosis or pneumonia compared with changes in nutritional and housing standards brought about as much by industrialisation and relative personal prosperity as by governmental action. In contemplating these events however we must not confuse population statistics with the enormous impact of medical advances on the survival prospects of individual patients, who must always be the doctor's first concern. This is classical social pathology. Less well documented are the psychological effects of industrialisation, urbanisation and the nuclear family on men and women. It seems that once man is sure of food and shelter his expectations usually rise continuously with each improvement in his lot.

As we saw in the last chapter, some people seek escape from the conflict between their expectations and their achievements by becoming a patient. This then is another example of social pathology, but the disease of rising expectations affects society as a whole as well as causing individual casualties. As a disease of society, it is known to us all as inflation.

The usual meaning of social pathology relates to diseases of individuals in which the main cause lies in the shortcomings or demands of society. These sociological factors are not necessarily as obvious as those which disgraced the Industrial Revolution. Stressful life events of all sorts including bereavement, moving home or changing or losing jobs can precipitate or exacerbate illness, not just depression but also streptococcal pharyngitis, rheumatoid arthritis and accidental trauma.

In the classical type of social pathology, i.e. disease due to socio-economic conditions the worst examples have as we have already seen in advanced societies been solved, firstly by social change and secondly by scientific discoveries. There were for example only 11 000 deaths from tuberculosis in the UK in 1971 compared with almost a quarter of a million deaths from heart disease.

This comparison is particularly interesting because a very large part of the death toll from diseases such as coronary thrombosis and carcinoma of the colon is associated with what we now regard as western standards of nutrition and hygiene, whereas death from infectious diseases used to be inversely related to the same factors. The rising mortality from 'Western' conditions such as ischaemic heart disease and bronchial carcinoma correlates so closely with the coincident decline in deaths from diseases of poverty that it is almost as if an ecological balance were being struck.

Affluence however is a relative term. Great Britain in the 1970's bears little resemblance to the grim Dickensian world of the mid-nineteenth century. Nevertheless age-corrected death rates from all causes, for virtually all individual diseases and also infant mortality, still show a strong inverse correlation with socio-economic class. For 1970/72, in social class I (e.g. the higher professionals) the standardised mortality ratio from all causes between the ages of 15-64 years was 77. For social class V (unskilled workers) it was 137, almost double. The corresponding figures for a disease of 'affluence', coronary heart disease, were 88 for social class I and 111 for social class V. As can be seen from Table 45.1 there is a continuous gradation through

Table 45.1 Mortality ratios of men in England and Wales between the ages of 15 and 64 years, in 1970-72, expressed by socio-economic group. Standardised mortality ratio for total male population = 100

Social class		Standardised Mortality Ratio	
		All causes of death	Coronary heart disease
I	(Professional)	77	88
II	(Employers, lesser professions)	81	91
III	(Non-manual workers)	99	114
III	(Skilled-manual workers)	106	107
IV	(Semi-skilled workers)	114	108
V	(Unskilled workers)	137	111

Table 45.2 Infant mortality in England and Wales by social class 1975-76. Expressed as deaths per 1000 live births

Social class		Neonatal (1st week of life)	Post-neonatal (1 week–2 yrs)
I		7.4	2.8
II		8.1	3.0
III	(non-manual workers)	8.5	3.3
III	(skilled manual workers)	9.5	4.2
IV		10.9	5.4
V		14.4	8.6

the social classes. The same is true of infant mortality (Table 45.2).

The sub-division of the population into social classes is one of the most crucial aspects of social pathology. The system in use is crude but valid. Various modifications have been proposed and the original social class III is often sub-divided into 'junior' non-manual workers and skilled manual workers. Whatever its shortcomings, it provides a very effective measure of the influence of socio-economic status on disease. The question of what causes the striking differences seen in Table 45.1 is one of the most interesting problems in social pathology. Social class correlates inversely with cigarette smoking, i.e. social class I has 29 per cent male smokers, class V 46 per cent. It correlates inversely with consumption of white bread, sugar and potatoes and positively with consumption of wholemeal bread and fruit. Social class I in 1977 consumed 33 oz. of fresh fruit per person per week, social class V only 17 oz. There is a dramatic inverse correlation between social class and participation in indoor and outdoor sports and games. In 1973 social class I had a participation index of 37 for outdoor sports and 18 for indoor games; social class V had corresponding figures of 8 and 4.

Not all health differences between classes can be explained by such easily measurable indices as smoking and diet. The incidence of depression in middle aged woman (p. 278) in inner cities was found by Brown to be 8 per cent in the middle class (I and II) and 25 per cent in classes IV and V. Brown attributes these differences to poorer marital communication, fewer opportunities for escape from young children and lower self-esteem.

There are many other expressions of increased morbidity (non-fatal illness) than depression. In men in the 45 to 64 year age group there is a dramatic rise in rates of acute and chronic sickness as the social class declines. This is reflected in a roughly corresponding rise in the consultation rate with general practitioners, as can be seen in Table 45.3.

In interpreting all these tables it would be wrong to assume that we are merely witnessing the effects of poverty. Only social class V can be said to be poor in the sense of nutritional and social deprivation. Most of the differences can be attributed to different occupations and styles of living. Some of these factors are unavoidable by those concerned, others might be altered by education. The dramatic inequalities between social class V and the rest of the populace are undoubtedly related to deprivation. Nevertheless even in a socialist utopia we could expect to find a proportion of the population whose health and life expectancy would be well below average because of their personal inadequacies.

There are other examples of the way medical advances seem to unmask new types of pathology. For many doctors the most difficult single clinical problem in their practice is the depressed, middle-aged married woman. Such a patient probably married young, is sufficiently well off to have no material worries but now finds that her children no longer need her and that she has made no intellectual or professional provision for such a day. It is not surprising that feeling baffled and useless she should accept the label of depressive illness. She may in fact be helped to deal with her situation by drugs which counteract her disabling depression but no one would pretend that they offer more than symptomatic relief. The point here is that until quite recent times only a minority of women survived the hazards of child birth, infection and poverty to reach middle age. Those that did would be unlikely to have avoided widowhood and re-marriage, or might merely be grateful and surprised to have outlived their contemporaries. In any event it is unlikely that psychological depression would have been a problem for this small band of survivors.

It is probably true of all societies that whatever the mores some

Table 45.3 Rates of acute and chronic sickness and consultations with general practitioners by social class, in men aged between 45–64 years, from 1974 to 76 in Great Britain. Acute illness is expressed as days per person per year, chronic illnesses rates per 1000. G.P. consultations as consultations per person per year

Socio-economic class		Acute illness	Chronic illness	General Practitioner Consultations
I		13	168	2.6
II		13	161	2.6
III	(non-manual workers)	21	261	4.0
III	(Skilled manual workers)	23	248	3.7
IV		21	275	4.0
V		29	380	5.4

individuals will feel so much at odds with them that they may seek refuge in illness. Doubtless in Victorian times there were many men and women whose sexual appetite differed from that prescribed by convention. Similarly, some people may nowadays be made to feel inadequate by the barrage of propaganda for continuous sexual activity. The remedy here is to disseminate the knowledge that as regards human behaviour normality is a purely mathematical term and that almost every human attribute, in its distribution in the population, follows the pattern of a Gaussian curve.

As we have said, the second type of social pathology involves the application to socio-economic problems of the methods of analyses that have proved successful in understanding disease. One of the cornerstones of pathology, the detection of a progressive failure of adaptation fits very obviously to the wage-price spiral of inflation. Pathology and natural selection are very closely linked, as this book should have made plain. Darwinian forces are at work in social pathology too but it would be unwise to draw premature conclusions as to where they are leading. The survival of society does not depend only upon economic success. As an example we can quote a country which becomes so successful that it finds its neighbours are too poor to buy its goods. For a time it will discover new customers but eventually adaptation will fail, unemployment will increase to unacceptable levels and security, prosperity and freedom may disappear overnight. In these changing circumstances survival of a society as defined by the preservation of law and of individual liberty may depend on characteristics such as excess of compassion and a lack of competitiveness which were disadvantageous in a different socio-economic setting.

A final contribution which pathology can perhaps make to sociology is to cast doubt on the science of predicting the future. A futurologist working in the fourteenth century would undoubtedly have prophesied the extinction of the populace by bubonic plague. He would have been justified, because increasing trade and population movement together with a trend to urbanisation all favoured the spread of this insect and rodent borne epidemic. Instead, after a flurry in the seventeenth century the plague become progressively less important and even now we are not sure why it behaved the way it did.

The history of disease suggests that all predictions based on present trends are almost certain to be wrong and that a belief in Divine intervention would be a more fruitful hypothesis than the view that current events have a predictive value for the future. In examining the direction in which society appears to be heading and its likely effects on his patients and himself the physician should recognise that the only certainty is that he can never be sure.

Bibliography

Dreitzel H P (ed) 1972 Family, marriage and the struggle of the sexes. MacMillan, New York

McKeown T 1977 The role of medicine. Oxford University Press, Oxford

Morris J N 1979 Social inequalities undiminished. Lancet 1: 87

The inequality of death. 1980 W.H.O Chronicle 34: 9

Tuckett D (ed) 1976 An introduction to medical sociology. Tavistock Publications, London

Worsley P (ed) 1974 Modern sociology. Penguin, Harmondsworth

Index of subjects

Note: Entries for illustrations and tables, due to their close proximity to the relevant text, are not italicised; main treatment of a subject is indicated by bold type.